FINGERS AND THUMBS

Toys and Activities for Children
with Hand–Function Problems

Roma Lear

Illustrated by Jill Hunter

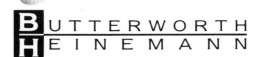

BUTTERWORTH
HEINEMANN

OXFORD   AUCKLAND   BOSTON   JOHANNESBURG   MELBOURNE   NEW DELHI

Butterworth-Heinemann
Linacre House, Jordan Hill, Oxford OX2 8DP
225 Wildwood Avenue, Woburn, MA 01801–2041
A division of Reed Educational and Professional Publishing Ltd

 A member of the Reed Elsevier plc group

First published 1999

British Library Cataloguing in Publication Data
Lear, Roma
 Fingers and thumbs: toys and activities for children with
 hand-function problems. – (Play can help)
 1. Hand – Abnormalities   2. Movement disorders in children
 3. Play therapy
 I. Title
 649.5'5'0873

ISBN 0 7506 2524 4

Composition by Genesis Typesetting, Rochester, Kent
Printed and bound in Great Britain by Martins The Printers, Berwick upon Tweed

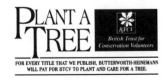

FOR EVERY TITLE THAT WE PUBLISH, BUTTERWORTH-HEINEMANN
WILL PAY FOR BTCV TO PLANT AND CARE FOR A TREE.

'Play Can Help' Series

FINGERS AND THUMBS

Books by the same author

In this series
Look at it This Way   ISBN 0 7506 3895 8

Also
Play Helps (Fourth Edition)   ISBN 0 7506 2522 8

Contents

Acknowledgements

My grateful thanks to Jill Norris who started the first special needs toy library in the UK and founded the National Association of Toy and Leisure Libraries. She inspired us all to learn so much about the value of play and toys.

I am also indebted to:

All the children who, over the years, have unwittingly supplied the material for this book.

All the parents and therapists who have shared their ideas with me for the benefit of other children. You will find their names scattered throughout the book. The royalties earned from their contributions will benefit the National Association of Toy and Leisure Libraries.

All my toy library friends and the staff at NATLL for their encouragement, suggestions and advice.

Jill Hunter for her delightful illustrations, and Stuart Wynn-Jones, Anita Jackson and Caroline Gould for supplementary pictures.

Ann Kirk for her good humoured and meticuluous editing.

And particularly to my husband, John, who has acted as critic and sounding board throughout the writing of this book.

Disclaimer

Every effort has been made to ensure that the information contained in this book is as accurate, informed and up-to-date as possible at the time of going to press. The author and publisher can neither be held liable for any errors or omissions, nor for any consequences of using inappropriately the toys and activities suggested.

Introduction to the 'Play Can Help' series

The toys and activities which make up the contents of this book come mainly from 'Play Helps – Toys and Activities for Children With Special Needs', fourth edition. That book is a collection of ideas relevant to children with widely differing play needs, and the toys and activities are arranged under the headings of the five senses. In the 'Play Can Help' series those which will be helpful to a child with a more specific disability have been collected together in one volume. A few ideas of general interest may overlap from one book to another, but plenty of new ideas specific to the group in question have been added.

The first volume in the series, 'Look at it This Way', is concerned with toys and play for children with a visual impairment. 'Fingers and Thumbs' is for children with hand-function problems. It is not intended to be a course in therapy. It is up to the reader to select appropriately from the large collection of ideas. Many of these have originated from my long association with the Kingston-upon-Thames Toy library—for children with special needs—or are ideas I dreamed up to amuse my own children. Over the years I have been privileged to know many professionals (physiotherapists, occupational therapists, teachers, play leaders, etc.), who have shared their expertise with me, and many parents who have 'put me in the picture' and helped me to see life through the eyes of their children. Many have contributed ideas which appear in the book under their names. The proportion of Royalties on these contributions will continue to be paid to the National Association of Toy and Leisure Libraries.

The toys are all home-made by someone, but not necessarily by you! Busy parents, carers and professionals may not have time or energy for such creativity—more is the pity—but, within a circle of family and friends, local clubs for retired people, sheltered workshops, etc., help may often be found. It might even be possible to start an Active Group. These are formed by people with a variety of skills between them who are willing to use their expertise to create 'one-off' toys for individual children. An Active Group operates from my house. Professionals (therapists, teachers, parents) and 'makers' meet once a term. Requests are made and the finished toys are collected at the next meeting. Cost of materials is met by the customer.

The toys in this book are described as *Instant*, (self explanatory—likely to be ephemeral) *Quick* (can be made in an evening and will probably last for long enough) or *Long-lasting* (may take a weekend to make, but will be much more child-resistant!). With every home-made toy the question of safety always arises. This is a burning issue for the toy trade too, yet I guess hardly a day passes without the Accident and Emergency Department of your local hospital having to help a child in trouble over a toy. Screws can work loose, wood can chip and splinter, seams split, and busy fingers soon work a tiny hole into a wide gap revealing stuffing and 'innards' which should have remained concealed. A toy, which may be perfectly safe for one child, may be disasterous in the hands of her friend. All adults caring for children with special needs must be extra vigilant and use common sense in massive doses. The alternative is to incarcerate the children in a bare padded room! While every care has been taken with regard to safety, it is up to adults to select appropriately for the children in question, for it is in the nature of childhood that a toy will be used in other ways than expected, and, if it is popular, it is likely to be loved to bits.

If you have never made a toy before (and you are in good company!), start with something simple—labelled *Instant* or *Quick*—which you feel will be appreciated by your child. Read the 'Before you begin' section for practical tips on safety and construction.

As you glance through the book you may say to yourself 'How simple! Why didn't I think of that?' or 'I used to do that as a child, but I had forgotten all about it.' This is my justification for including some elementary and traditional ideas. They give excellent play value, are new to the children—and there really is no need to reinvent the wheel!

For the benefit of the book's users, the toys are categorised under common hand movements—anything from 'Holding on' to 'Doing up Buttons'. Each section begins with a list of its contents. The easier ideas come first. There is also an opening section on 'Making play possible'. This may be particularly helpful for children with mobility problems or who have unsteady movements.

The book is all about having fun—with only a whiff of therapy! It is intended to be used rather as a collection of cookery recipes—not read from cover to cover but dipped into now and then. I hope you will find plenty to tickle your palate!

July 1999   Roma Lear

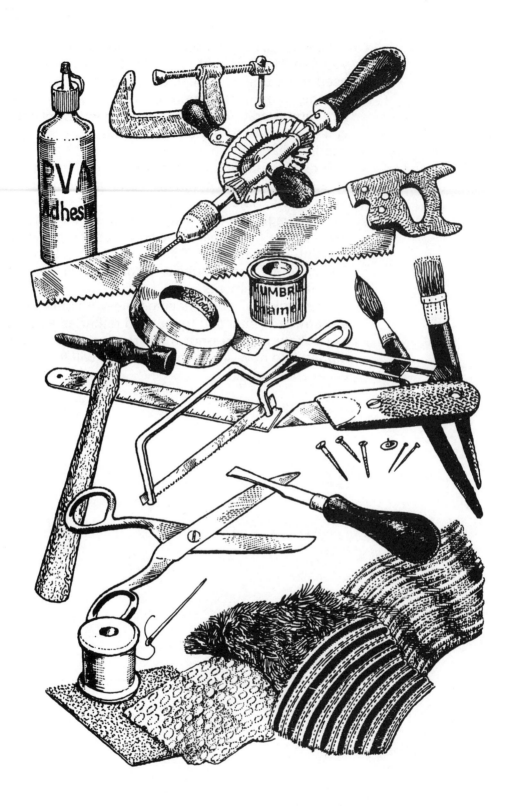

Before you begin

I hope you will find many toys in this book that will be both fun and a help to the child you have in mind. Before you start to make any toy, consider the safety factor carefully. One toy may be a winner with one child, but be bad news for another. Remember the child with a voracious appetite and strong, busy fingers mentioned in the Introduction who even now may be waiting his turn in the Accident and Emergency Department of your local Hospital! Small, fragile, or badly-made toys are not for him (or her!) Other children can play perfectly safely and have fun with a small or ephemeral toy. After all, they are doing it all the time when left to their own devices and play with whatever comes to hand—a ruler and an elastic band, matches, knives . . . all fraught with danger in the wrong hands! So SAFETY FIRST. Consider the habits of the child **and his neighbours** as you select your toy. You are the one in charge!

If you decide to make a *long-lasting* toy, use the best materials available. The result of your efforts will look good, be a pleasure to make, and will last longer.

- Use birch plywood or Medium Density Fibreboard for wooden toys. Both sand down well and you can avoid splinters and rough edges.
- New fabric is much stronger than some which has been through the wash many times. Use it double or back it with calico for extra strength.
- Pay special attention to seams and fastening off. Stitch them twice and oversew the edges to prevent fraying and splitting.
- Sew buttons on very securely with strong button thread.
- PVA adhesive is excellent for sticking paper, thin card or fabric, and is watersolvent. If you want a stronger bond, use a glue in a tube. Read the directions on the tube first to make sure the adhesive is non-toxic and suitable for the job.
- All paints and felt pens bearing the CE mark and sold as suitable for school use will be non-toxic. Humbrol enamel, sold in small tins for painting models, etc., comes in bright colours, dries quickly and is safe to use on toys.
- Polyurethane varnish is non-toxic when dry. Two or three coats will form a tough protective covering and make the toy washable.
- Polyester fibre for soft toys is sold at craft shops, upholstery departments, etc. The bag should be labled 'suitable for toy making' and bear the CE safety mark.

The great advantage of making your own toys—apart from the fun of it—is that they can be personalised to suit their user. You may need to make a toy heavy, or light, simple (make fewer pieces than suggested) or more complicated (increase the number). A toy can be thrown together as a five-minute wonder, be fun for a while, but soon end up in the bin, or it can be constructed with care to become a treasured posession and last for years. I believe there is room in the day for both. Obviously circumstances alter cases, and the choice is always yours!

STRENGTHENING TOYS WITH PAPIER MÂCHÉ

Perhaps the making of papier mâché is a technique new to you. If that is so, and you would like to try it, read on for some handy hints, which should help you achieve really good results.

First, some general thoughts on the versatility of the technique. It seems strange that a material as floppy as a piece of newspaper can, with the help of flour-and-water paste, be laminated to make a substance as strong as wood. The cost is minimal! In this book, papier mâché has been used to strengthen a thin cardboard box and convert it into a virtually child-proof toy—as with the Slither Box, p. 50. With the Milk Bottle Monster (p. 106), the same technique has been used to attach the cardboard spine and tail trimmings to the milk bottle. Once the paper and paste have been applied and left to dry, the trimmings are held firmly in place by the layers of paper. As an added advantage, the greasy surface to the plastic milk bottle is covered and can now be painted.

Newspaper can also be used as a modelling medium. It is torn into tiny pieces, soaked in a bucket of water until the pieces start to fall apart, squeezed as dry as possible, then thoroughly mixed with stiff flour and water paste. The result is a grey and soggy mess! However, this is easy to convert into sausages, bananas, apples, or potatoes (etc!) for shop play. More proficient modellers can form the mixture into faces, haystacks and hedges for farm layouts or a hundred and one other 3D items.

In countries where trees and money are scarce, furniture—including made-to-measure chairs and tables for children with disabilities—are made from cardboard, newspaper and paste. There are simple techniques which ensure a safe and robust result. If you are interested in using papier mâché for such large items, contact the addresses for APT (Alternative Paper Technology) on p. 8.

The paper

- Always use unglazed paper. It absorbs the paste better.

- Before you begin, collect some 'normal' newspaper and some of a different colour—say the pink of *The Financial Times* or coloured pages from a children's comic. Using two colours makes it easy to apply the layers of paper evenly. It is obvious where you have been, and so 'holidays' and weak spots can be avoided.
- Mass produced paper has a 'grain' and will easily tear into a straight strip if you tear with the grain. Sometimes this runs horizontally across the page, sometimes vertically. It is easy to find out which is the right direction for *your* pages by ripping one from top to bottom, then from side to side. One way you will get a neat, straight tear, the other way the tear will be unpredictable.
- If you are working on a large surface, such as reinforcing the Card Posting Box (p. 79), you can speed up the process by applying sheets of newspaper three at a time. Having established the lie of the grain, cover one sheet with paste. Cover it with another sheet—grain in the same direction as the first, of course—paste it, and finish off the triple-decker sandwich with the third sheet. Now all three layers can be torn into strips at the same time and be applied to the toy as one. Next, cover the surface with a layer of contrasting paper, then another layer of 'triple decker'. If neccessary, repeat the process until the papier mâché covering is thick enough.
- The final layer should be applied in cheap white unglazed paper. This will cover up the news print. Alternatively, you can give the finished (dry) toy a coat of white paint before you paint it properly.

Applying the paper

- Always *tear* the paper. This gives it a ragged edge and helps it to blend with the next piece. If you cut it, you will get a hard line round the edge of each piece, and this makes for a less smooth finish.
- Make sure the paper is well pasted, but not too soggy. If the paste is not applied evenly—either to the part of the toy you are working on, or to the paper—there

will be dry patches which will not stick properly. If too much paste is used, the toy will take seemingly for ever to dry out.

- For speed, apply the paper in strips. This is easy on a flat surface, but for curves and corners the strips must be torn into smaller pieces. Take particular care to put extra layers of paper at corners and weak spots (such as where the spine and tail join onto the Milk Bottle Monster).
- Make sure each piece of paper is properly stuck down and slightly overlapping its neighbour. There should be no bubbles, wrinkles or unpasted edges.
- The number of layers applied depends on how strong the toy needs to be. It is a good idea to put on (say) five layers. Leave them to dry out. Test the toy for strength. Does it dent? Do the applied parts wobble? If the answer is 'yes', it's back to more layers and another overnight pause for them to dry out.
- Drying out has been mentioned several times . It is essential to be patient over this. If you paint too quickly, the result will be patchy and disappointing.
- Finally, protect the toy with at least two coats of polyurethane varnish. This makes it spongeable and helps the corners to remain unscuffed.

Mixing the paste

- 1 heaped tablespoon of plain flour
- A little cold water—about 100 ml—enough to mix the flour to a smooth paste
- About 400 ml of *boiling water*
- A Pyrex jug

Put the flour in the jug. Very gradually add the cold water, squashing out all the lumps, until the mixture looks like cream. Stir continuously and pour in the boiling water until you have made a pint of paste (500 ml). For safety's sake, it is best for one person to hold the jug and stir, while a second person pours in the boiling water. This is NOT a job for children.

As you add the boiling water, the flour will partly cook. The mixture becomes thicker and more translucent. Once it has cooled, it is ready for use.

SOME MATERIALS USED

Bells	From a pet or craft shop or in packets of 50 from Edu-play.
Buddies or Sticky Fixers	From any stationers.
Button thread	A strong, twisted thread necessary for sewing on buttons.
Dowel rod in pine or ramin (stronger)	Made in various thicknesses. From wood yards and DIY stores.
Dycem	A plastic material with special non-slip qualities. Available in various shapes and thicknesses. Can be ordered from the Dispensary at Boots the Chemists or from Nottingham Rehab.
Fish grit	Normally used at the bottom of an acquarium, but useful for washable bean bags, noisemakers, etc. From a pet shop.
Humbrol enamel	Sold in small pots for painting models, etc. Non-toxic, bright colours, dries quickly. Widely available.
Magnetic tape	A strip (or sheet) of pliable, magnetised, rubber-like plastic with an adhesive backing. It can be cut to size with scissors. Peel off the backing and apply to toys as required. From Educational Suppliers and may also be found in High Street shops.
Plastic foam	NEVER use uncovered. This material is not suitable for children who 'pick'. In the right situation it is useful for making large, light bricks, etc. From shops dealing in upholstery materials, street markets.
Polyurethane varnish	Non-toxic when dry(!) Use two or more coats for a tough, wipeable skin for a wooden toy. From any shop selling paint.

PVA adhesive   Non-toxic. Watersolvent if not set. If hardened, will peel off. Dries transparent. (If accidentally spilt on clothing, put it in the freezer! It becomes brittle and will flake off.) Can be diluted with cold water. (Hot water will set it.) From any stationer, Early Learning Centre, etc.

Velcro   Comes in circles and strips. I have found the circles in two sizes—Velcro Spots, and Velcoins, which are slightly larger. Used in upholstery, dressmaking, etc. Available in the High Street, or in a wider selection from Nottingham Rehab.

SOME USEFUL ADDRESSES

For some people living in rural areas or with heavy demands on their time, personal shopping is not always an easy option. Here is a short list of mail-order firms, correct at the time of going to press.

The Craft Depot
1, Canvin Court, Somerton Business Park,
Somerton, Somerset TA11 6SB
Tel: 01458 274 727
For a wide range of plastic canvas, touch'n play music buttons, squeakers, etc.

Edu-play
Units H and I, Vulcan Business Centre,
Vulcan Road, Leicester LE5 3EB
Tel: 01533 525 827
For bells, difraction paper and a selection of unusual toys.

Hope Education
Orb Mill, Huddersfield Road,
Oldham, Lancashire OL4 2ST
Tel: 01616 336 611
For magnetic tape, and other useful items like blank dice, scissors with unusual grips, etc.

Just Fillings
Dept. PC, 1, Beechroyd, Pudsey,
West Yorkshire LS28 8BH
Tel: 01274 691 965
For a selection of polyester fibre.

NES Arnold
Ludlow Hill Road, West Bridgford,
Nottingham NG2 6HG
Tel: 01159 452 201
Also for magnetic tape, etc.

Nottingham Rehab
Address as for NES Arnold
Tel: 01159 452 345
For Dycem in various shapes and grades, a wide range of Velcro, special scissors, etc.

Some toy mail-order companies

John Adams Trading Company Limited
32, Milton Park, Abingdon,
Oxfordshire OX14 4RT
Tel: 01235 833 066
Particularly for a wide range of
reasonably-priced craft kits.

Escor Toys
Elliott Road, Bournemouth BH11 8JP
Tel: 01202 591 181
For a range of peg toys.

Rompa
Goyt Side Road, Chesterfield S40 2PH
Tel: 01246 211 777

Step by Step Ltd.
Lavenham Road,
Beeches Trading Estate,
Yate, Bristol BS37 5QX
Tel: 01454 320 200
For toys for up to about eight years of age
and many materials for children's
creativity.

TFH
76, Barracks Road, Sandy Lane Industrial
Estate, Stourport-on-Severn,
Worcestershire DY 13 9QB
Tel: 01299 827 820

Some more useful addresses

Anything Left Handed
18, Avenue Road,
Belmont, Sutton,
Surrey SM2 6JD
Tel: 0181 770 3722
This is the mail-order address.
There is also a shop in London at
57, Brewer Street, W1R 3FB which could
be useful for older children.
Tel: 0171 437 3910

Intermediate Technology Publications Ltd
103–105 Southampton Row,
London WC1B 3HH
Tel: 0171 436 9761
For *'Appropriate Paper-Based Technology'*
(APT). A Manual. Bevill Packer.

*National Association of Toy and Leisure
Libraries*
68, Churchway, London NW1 1LT
Tel: 0171 387 9692
For the address of your nearest toy library,
and an excellent publication 'Switch to Play'
which tells you all you need to know about
switch toys. It includes a long list of
suppliers, a book list, and advice on
computers and communication aids.

Making play possible

EVERYONE CARING FOR CHILDREN WITH SPECIAL NEEDS knows how difficult it can often be to keep toys within reach of the child who is playing with them— and, occasionally, out of reach of the one who shouldn't be! All children who, for whatever reason, are unable to choose and fetch their own toys will need help before they can start to play.

Cot and pram toys are easily bought for babies. Such toys will neither appeal nor be appropriate for older children who, because of their disabilities, may still continue to spend part of their time in a cot. They need their own playthings adapted for cot use. Other children are able to sit in a chair, but their hand function may be very limited. Perhaps they have jerky, uncoordinated movements—without help their toys can be swept to the floor or knocked out of reach. And so the list can continue.

If your child has difficulty in reaching or retaining her toys, read on. Help may be among the tried and tested ideas that follow.

KEEPING TOYS WITHIN REACH

Suspending toys for children who are lying down

The following devices should be positioned within easy reach of the children's hands so that they can biff, grab, grasp and let go as they please.

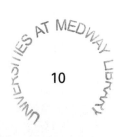

An Elastic Luggage Strap

Instant

This has strong hooks on both ends and can be hung across the cot, so that the child can biff and grab the toys that dangle from it. It can easily be removed when the cot side needs lowering. It should be *slightly* stretched between the cot rails, so it is wise to measure before buying. Hang some toys with tape or string, but use elastic for others so that, when they are pulled and released, they will bob about.

An Elastic Washing Line

Instant

Jeanette Maybanks

Here is an easy, but effective, way of suspending toys at any height. The brainwave came from a busy Mum who wanted to amuse her baby while he was still at the precrawling stage and floorbound on a rug. The idea could be used to hang toys within reach of any child who needs to play in a similar position. Just hang a length of elastic between two suitable points—the rungs of chairs might do. At intervals along it, attach strong bulldog clips. (These are obtainable from large stationers and office equipment suppliers.) As the name suggests, these clips grip very firmly and will withstand a fair amount of tugging. From the clips, dangle any old thing, perhaps a handkerchief, or a fluorescent sock with a rattle in the toe, a soft toy on a piece of ribbon or a glove with a little bell in a finger.

A Plastic Garden Chain

Instant
(and long-lasting)

Here is another way of stringing toys in a row, either for a child in a cot, or for one lying on the floor. The chain looks attractive and, of course, is very strong—and washable! When it is firmly fixed in position, simply tie the toys to the links, position the child comfortably and let her have a go.

Goal Posts

Long-lasting

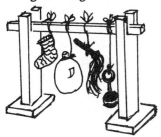

This idea is borrowed from the football pitch. A child can lie between the posts and reach all the delights that dangle from the crossbar. The posts are slotted (or fixed with brackets) into sturdy feet so that the whole frame is very stable. The crossbar rests in grooves cut in the top of the posts and, at the end of playtime, the whole contraption can be taken apart for easy storage.

A Hotch Potch of Toys to Biff, Grab or Pull

Instant

Suggested by
Christine Cousins,
Judy Denziloe,
Margaret Gilmore,
Alison Harland, Lilli
Nielson, Linda Bennet
School, Fiona Priest,
RNIB Advisers,
Jean Vant.

Select as appropriate.
- Balloons. Sausage-shaped ones are easier to hit. (To minimise the risk of a balloon popping, do not over inflate.) A few grains of rice inside, or a small bell or two, make them even more exciting.
- A bunch of ribbons or non-fray strips of material.
- Any plastic bottle with a handle, and something (safe) inside it to rattle. Fix the lid on with a dab of plastic glue, e.g. U-Hu.
- A sock with something tactile in the toe—such as a rattle, fir cone or squeaky toy. Stitch across the top and attach a string.
- A string of large buttons, perhaps with a bell (from the pet shop) added here and there.
- A plastic sweet jar with something interesting in it such as coloured cotton reels, ping pong balls or cat balls with a bell inside.
- An 'octopus' made from coloured tights stuffed with newspaper and tied together at the top.
- A danglement made from pipe insulation tubing.
- Hang a soft toy. Perhaps suspend it from a length of elastic, so that it will bob about if pulled and released.
- See if a plastic baby mirror appeals. This is large and shiny and has convenient holes round the edge from which to hang it.
- Hang up a *bunch* of rattles—much easier for a child to focus on and biff or grab than a single one.
- Thread coloured cotton reels on a string. Join the ends together to form a loop.
- Use the lid from a treacle tin with a small hole punched near the rim. This lid is strong, shiny and has a well-turned edge. To make its rotations more dramatic, stick a circle of brightly-coloured Fablon or some stickers on one side.
- Make a tassel from a few lengths of string. Thread some large buttons on each string. Tie a knot below each button and leave a space before threading on the next one. When the child pulls a string or swipes at the lot, the buttons should click together.
- Use an empty bag from a wine box. Inflate it and, perhaps, put some adhesive stickers on it.
- Look around the kitchen for likely objects. Even a wooden spoon could be a winner.

See also
Bamboo Mobile, p. 65
Ship's Bell Rattle, p. 67
Grab Bags, p. 56
Amorphous Beanbag, with strings attached, p. 57
Manx Feely Cushion, with strings attached, p. 57

For children playing on the floor

Instant

Pam Courtney,
Deputy Head Teacher,
St Anne's School

A child with multiple disabilities is sure to have great difficulty in keeping his toys within reach. He may have limited or uncontrolled movements, perhaps combined with poor sight or hearing. It is not surprising that, with all these problems, he may soon lose interest in his play. If he pushes his toys away with an involuntary movement, there they will stay—out of reach—out of sight—and probably out of mind. The child is left with nothing to do until someone notices his plight.

Pam has suggested two simple and instant ways to overcome this problem:

1. Playing on a Sloping Surface

If the child is playing on the floor and lying on one side, a sheet of hardboard can be placed between him and the wall. The far edge of the hardboard is raised (prop it up on the telephone directory!) so that when toys are pushed away they will slide down and back to him.

2. Playing in a Baby Bath

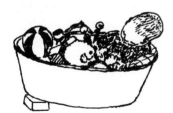

For a small child who is able to sit up, a baby bath with one end slightly raised makes a good 'child and toy container'. The high sides of the bath also help to keep toys to hand. Pam has found that, for some children, it is better to put plenty of toys in the bath—not just one or two. This bonanza cannot be ignored and should tempt the child to investigate, and play. As an alternative to a baby bath, you might use a plastic laundry basket. This has the added advantage that toys can be strung across it or tied to the sides—useful if the child might otherwise end up sitting on them. For ways of keeping toys to hand for older children playing on the floor, search through the section on bed play below. The problems can be similar.

For children in bed

A Play Cushion

Quick

Susan Harvey and
Ann Hales-Tooke

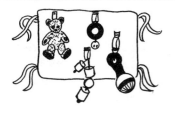

In the early days of play in hospital, these pioneering play specialists devised unusual cushions for very young patients who needed nursing in oxygen tents. In this situation the children continually lost their toys among the folds of the tent. To overcome the problem, hospital pillows, already encased in washable plastic, were given attractive, removable outer covers. Rings or loops were firmly attached to one side, and tie strings to the other. Rattles, soft toys, etc. were attached to the loops as needed, and the tie strings fixed the cushions securely to the cot bars—to avoid any danger of them falling onto the children.

Method
- Use new material (for strength.) Make sure it is washable.
- Choose a plain colour. The toys show up better.
- Keep the strings attached to the toys fairly short to avoid tangling.
- Remember to hold the child's interest by changing the toys now and then.

A Play Table for Bed or Floor

Quick

Alison Wisbeach,
Occupational
Therapist

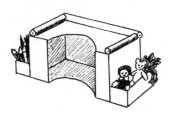

Children in hospital are provided with special tables to fit over their beds. For the child who is nursed at home, Alison has thought up a quickly-made play table. She begins with a sturdy cardboard box, (e.g. one from the Off Licence) and cuts a knee hole in one side. Plastic foam pipe wrap is glued to the top edges of the other three sides, making a retaining wall to prevent toys from falling off. Finally, she glues empty shoe boxes to each side to hold toys, felt pens, paper, etc. Thus equipped, the child should have everything to hand for a happy play time.

A Revolving Play Tidy

*Instant
(and long-lasting)*

One of our little toy library members was quite a worry to us until, one day, we had a sudden brainwave, and came up with a simple answer to her play problem! Imagine Mandy, a lively three-year-old, sitting in her made-to-measure wheelchair with its tray in position in front of her. Because of her disability, she had unusually short arms, so only half of the area of the tray was of use to her. Toys that strayed beyond the middle were out of reach. Tough! Our simple solution was to provide her with a cake icing turntable—from the kitchen department of a High Street shop—and we found we had instantly extended her play area. The turntable could also be placed on a table to one side of the wheelchair. In this position, it could hold pieces of jigsaw or perhaps doll's house furniture—whatever was the toy of the moment. Mandy could help herself to the piece required and transfer it to her tray. The next step was to provide her with a Reacher (*see* below) and she was well away!

If you have ever used a turntable when playing Scrabble, you will see other advantages in this simple device. It can come in handy when playing small board games. With a little skill in carpentry, it can even be custom-made in wood. To meet a particular need, the circular revolving surface could be made larger, or even square. A rim could be attached to the lip to stop small items falling off. (Another barrier might be needed to prevent objects straying towards the centre and out of reach.)

For older children with limited reach, the same idea can be used to make storage space for pencils, rubbers, rulers, felt pens, scissors, glue . . . or what you will. Simply attach some containers of different sizes to the surface of the turntable (screw or glue!) and, with a flick of the wrist, the child can bring everything within range.

A Reacher

Quick

Alison Wisbeach

Some of us are familiar with the reachers available commercially for adults. (By squeezing a handle at one end of a rod, a claw at the other can be made to pick up dropped objects.) Smaller versions are available for children, but not all can manage the controlled movements they require. Alison has come to the rescue again with this simple reacher. She makes it from a length of dowel, drills a small hole in one end and screws in a large cup hook. With this cheap and handy little device, straying toys can easily be hooked back into play.

15

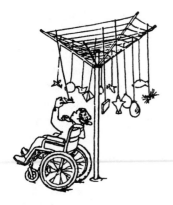

Of course, the length and thickness (and con-
sequently the weight) of the dowel can be adjusted to
suit the user. If the dowel is thin and likely to split, bind
round the cup hook end with button thread or thin
string.

For children in wheelchairs

**The Whirly Clothes
Line**

Instant

When the warm weather is here (and the washing has
dried,) why not use the whirly line as an outdoor toy
holder? The fact that it revolves adds to its attraction,
and a determined child can tug his way to the toy of his
choice.

**A Three-sided Clothes
Horse**

Quick

Leicester Toy Library

One day a very tiny three-year-old girl with both
physical and learning difficulties visited the Leicester
Toy Library. Much of her time was spent in her extra
small wheelchair, so her Mum was looking for suitable
toys that she could watch and perhaps reach out and
touch. An ingenious member of the toy library staff
realised that the doll's clothes horse from a laundry play
set would fit snugly round the wheel chair. It could be
tied to the arms to make it stable, and all sorts of toys
could be hung from the rails. The cage and bells from a
roller rattle was fixed to the top one. This turned out to
be the most popular item, for everyone passing by was
tempted to give the cage a whirl—much to the delight
of the little girl. Toys like pull-string music boxes, rattles,
and paper toys that moved in the draught were hung
from other rails. Using this simple, ready-made frame,
the child was surrounded on three sides by attractive
playthings, easily changed for others when they no
longer appealed. Safe and happy behind her toy frame,
she could still watch everything that was going on
around her.

This idea, but using a normal, domestic-sized, clothes
horse as a toy holder—or perhaps as somewhere to
hang frequently needed items—might also be helpful to
any child in a wheelchair.

For children playing at a table

A Tabletop Necklace

Quick

Mrs Crane,
Teacher,
The Manor School

Tying toys to a necklace for a child to wear is obviously not a good idea, because of the risk of it tightening round his neck, but to make a string of playthings which can be looped over a tabletop is a safe way of keeping toys within reach.

The first tabletop necklace I came across was made in desperation by a teacher in a school for children with severe learning difficulties. In her group were several lively lads, and one who was not able to move from his wheelchair. This boy was quiet and gentle. His favourite occupation was to shake and rattle plastic toys. Unfortunately, his class mates often took a fancy to his playthings and grabbed them from him, leaving him very upset, (naturally!). His teacher came up with this answer. She collected up all his favourite toys. Then, using long strips of fabric, she made a plait. She laid this over his play table. Once the ends were tied together to form a loop, the plait could not slide off. The next step was to spread out the toys and tie them with tape at intervals along the plait. The boy could now sit at the table and pull the necklace towards him until he reached the toy of his choice. He might go for a large plastic ring with strings of buttons attached, a plastic car, a pair of plastic scissors, a trainer ball with holes in it and a bell inside, a string of large beads, a bunch of keys or one of the various rattles. At last he could enjoy his favourite activity in uninterrupted peace.

A very simple way of using this idea is to buy a suitable length of plastic chain, obtainable from a garden centre, etc. Loop the chain over the table top, join the ends together, and tie toys to the links.

A Tabletop Play Corner

Quick

Judy Denziloe,
Project Coordinator,
Planet

How can you help a seated child keep her toys conveniently on the top of the table when her jerky movements tend to sweep them to the floor? Judy uses a sizeable square cardboard carton from the supermarket. She cuts it diagonally in half and takes one piece to make the triangular play space. Toys can be played with on the floor of the box and the high sides will prevent them from being pushed out of reach. If appropriate, you can make holes in the sides and dangle

17

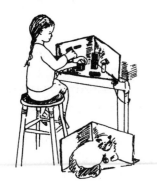

toys from them. The tabletop play corner is certain to need stabilising. Perhaps sticking it to the table with masking tape or Blu-tac will be sufficient. Otherwise, try wedging it in place with something heavy—the telephone directory? sandbags? a covered brick? or make a few holes at the bottom of the sides and tie the whole affair down securely.

For children who tend to scatter their toys

A Picture Frame

Instant

Jenny Buckle,
Play Leader and Parent

It is so easy for toys with many small pieces—such as Lego bricks or Play People with all their accessories—to end up scattered all over the tabletop and possibly out of reach. Put them inside a picture frame and the problem could be solved!

Magnetic Tape and a Metal Playboard

Quick

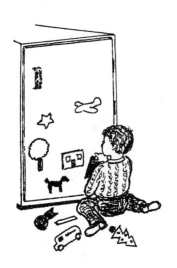

This method of keeping toys within reach can be fun for all children. But it is particularly helpful for those with jerky movements and poor hand-eye co-ordination.

Play pieces with the magnetic tape (or magnets) attached to them will stick to the board until the child chooses to move them. He has *time* to aim for the pieces he wishes to move.It is even possible to make the adhesion light or firm, according to the amount of magnetic tape that is applied. On the down side, of course, any sort of magnet is totally indigestible so the ideas suggested below are *only* for older children of known habits who have no desire to pick off the magnets and eat them!

Magnetic tape can be obtained from educational suppliers (p. 7) and can sometimes be found in High Street shops. With the current craze for making fridge magnets, a shop selling craft items will also stock disc and bar magnets, which are useful for heavier items.

A metal playboard is essential. You might already have a nicely framed playboard from a toy shop, (usually sold complete with magnetic letters, numbers and shapes). If not, your child can manage perfectly well with a large baking tray or the door of the fridge, or even the front of the radiator in summer time when the heat is turned off.

Years ago, when I was working as the toymaker at a hospital for people with severe learning difficulties, I used a panel from an unwanted gas cooker! This was standing in my neighbour's garden, awaiting disposal by the refuse collector. With my neighbour's approval, I unscrewed a side, protected the edges with some layers of strong plastic tape, and, (for free!) we had a splendid space for magnetic play!

Push-together puzzles lend themselves beautifully to this form of play. They have non-interlocking pieces which are just 'pushed together' in the right order to make up the picture. In the toy library of the hospital mentioned above, we had an ancient and unattractive metal cupboard, which I brightened up with several small push-together puzzles. On Friday evenings I would muddle them up ready for our Monday morning visitors. Over the weekend the cleaner would amuse herself by putting them all back together again. She must have found them irresistible!

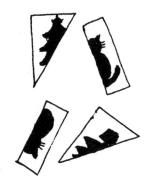

For a *quick* push-together puzzle, all you need is a Christmas Card. Stick the front to the back to make it stiffer. Wait for the glue to dry, then, with a wiggly line, cut the card into pieces—perhaps just two for a beginner, more for a child who is used to jigsaws. Apply magnetic tape to the backs of all the pieces. A friend makes similar (larger) puzzles using the brightly-coloured pictures on toy boxes made from thick card.

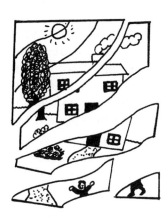

For *long-lasting* puzzles use ply. A picture merely stuck on may be 'picked' and the puzzle soon ruined. It is best to paint the picture directly onto the wood. With a fret saw cut wavy lines to divide the picture into the number of pieces you want and finally give it protective coats of polyurethane varnish.

More Magnetic Toys

Quick

Deborah Jaffé,
Toy Designer

Way back in 1975, Deborah Jaffé wrote a delightful little book called *Magnetic Board Toys*. It was published by the then Toy Libraries Association (now the National Association of Toy and Leisure Libraries) and sadly is no longer in print. Deborah has given me permission to pass on some of her ideas:

● From 4 mm ply or thick card, make a selection of shapes—squares, circles, rectangles, triangles.

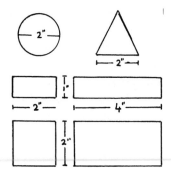

Colour them—acrylic paint is best, but poster paint or felt pens will do. It is wise to protect the painted surface with a coat of polyurethane varnish or cover it with clear sticky-backed plastic. Cut squares from the magnetic tape and stick them to the back of each shape. Several small squares of magnetic tape are better than one large one—or even a strip—because the adhesion to the metal board will be better. (We have already established that these toys are not for children who like to 'pick'!) In play, the shapes can be sorted into groups by shape or colour or used to make patterns or pictures.

● You can give a new lease of life to wooden animal templates normally used for drawing round. After much use, they can become well scribbled over and messy. Paint one side and add squares of magnetic tape to the other, and you have the makings of a farm or zoo. Using ply or thick card, cut out extra shapes for farm buildings, hay stacks, trees, hedges, gates, etc.

● Make a 'Creepy Crawly'. Consult the diagrams and take your pick.

Each one is made from two pieces of material, with strips of magnetic tape sandwiched in between. Choose lightweight material such as cotton, voile, poplin, or nylon. Indicate the eyes on the top piece. These can be snap-on safety eyes (from a craft shop), buttons (firmly attached), felt (stuck and stitched), or

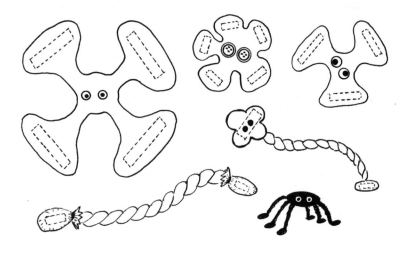

embroidered. On the bottom piece, stitch magnetic tape to the *inside* of the feet. (See dotted lines on the diagram.) Put the pieces right sides together and pin. Stitch most of the way round the edge, leaving a gap for turning. Turn right side out and close the gap (oversew).

- A creepy crawly snake or a worm can be made from a short length of piping cord—say 15 cm (6"). Sew magnetic tape to the ends. Cover the tape with little bags of material.

  Enlarge the snake /worm idea and make a spider with six feet. Use three slightly longer pieces of piping cord. Make the magnetic feet first—one at each end of the cord—before it tends to unwind. Overlap the cords at the middle and stitch them together. Splay out the legs for realism! Make a body from two ovals of black felt and top stitch them together to cover the cords where they intersect. Sew on beads for eyes or indicate them with French knots.

Playing in a Meat Tin or Cat Litter Tray

Either of these make good toy containers, and might be particularly helpful to a child lying on her tummy, over a wedge.

For children playing in the car

A Play Pinny

Quick

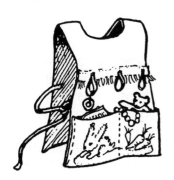

Over the years our toy library at Kingston-upon-Thames has been supplying pinnies of an appropriate size to children with visual or hand function problems. Toys tied to the loops on the front of this useful little cover-up cannot be dropped or pushed out of reach. Other toys, felt pens, etc. can be kept in the pocket at the bottom. On a long journey, a play pinny can be a boon to any small child strapped in his safety seat, possibly with no-one beside him to retrieve dropped playthings. The pinny ensures that child and toys stay together!

Materials
- A strip of reversible cotton (or similar) fabric, about the width of the child's shoulders. Length will depend on the size of the child, but a metre should be ample.

● Bias binding for the neck.
● Tape—for the toy loops and the side ties.

Method

Hem the raw edge at the bottom of the strip of fabric and turn it up. Tack this potential pocket at the sides. Fold the fabric in half. On the fold, cut out a modest hole for the child's head. (You can always enlarge it!) Try it on the model for size—too small and it will be a struggle to put on, too large and the pinny will be a sloppy fit. Neaten the neck edge with bias binding. Decide where the loops for attaching the toys will go. Mark the place with pins. Sew a strip of tape behind the pins. This reinforces the fabric, for the loops will have to withstand a fair amount of pulling and tweaking. Stitch the loops on firmly. Remove the pins, and hem the sides of the pinny including the pocket. Attach tapes at about the child's waist level. When the pinny is in use and these are tied with a bow, they will prevent it from rucking up or flapping about. Machine a row of stitches down the centre of the pocket to divide it into two, one side for each hand. Now all that is needed are some little surprises to hide in the pockets, (crunchy paper or a fir cone?) and some suitable toys to tie to the loops of tape (rattle, teether, soft toy?) Happy journeys!

SOME WAYS OF ADAPTING TOOLS AND TOYS FOR INDIVIDUAL NEEDS

Handles

Too short
● For sand-pit or gardening tools, search at the garden centre for lightweight tools (intended for elderly or disabled gardeners). These tools have an extending attachment that can be fitted to the handles.
● For pencils, saw off a suitable length of bamboo garden cane, sandpaper any rough edges and wedge the pencil inside the hollow centre.
● Paint brushes with long handles are obtainable at good toy shops or educational suppliers p. 7).

Too Long
- Cut them down or find a smaller equivalent, e.g. make-up brushes can be used for painting.
- Diary pencils or those used by Bridge players are short and thin.

Too Thin
- Pad them out with layers of rubber bands.
- Bandage tightly with strips of rag.
- Wind round with plastic foam and tie firmly.
- Poke a paint brush or pencil through the holes in a plastic golf practice ball.
- Use bicycle handle bar grips.
- Consult your therapist and buy specially shaped handles from a medical supplier.

Suggested by Jenny Buckle, The Disabled Living Foundation, Alison Wisbeach and R.L.

Inset Puzzles: Alternative Ways of Removing and Replacing the Pieces

Most manufacturers now offer a range of inset tray puzzles with knobs attached to each inset piece. For some children these certainly make the puzzle easier to manipulate, but they may not be the answer for those who cannot bring their fingers together in a 'tripod grip'. Often a small DIY addition to a commercial puzzle can turn a session of frustration into one of achievement. Here are four alternatives to knobs. The illustration shows an example of each.

1. Raise up all the inserted pieces
Cut out an identical shape in plywood, or thick card, and stick it to the bottom of the original piece. This will now stand proud of the tray and can be handled by grasping it round the edge.

2. Screw a plasticised cup hook into each inset piece
If this protrudes through to the underside, file it flat and smooth. This idea dates from the early days of toy libraries when Audrey Stevenson, an eminent and ingenious toy designer, found that by using this simple device some children with severe hand-function problems could manage to hook out the pieces and then replace them in their correct recesses. Being slender, the cup hooks hardly obscure the picture—as can happen when large knobs are attached.

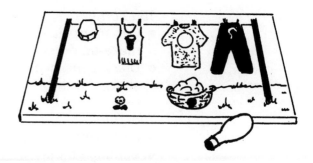

3. Insert a plastic golf tee into each piece.
This makes a fairly unobtrusive knob. It can be just the right shape for a child with small hands to grasp easily. Drill right through the inset piece and countersink a small depression on the underside. Poke the tee through the hole so that the tip protrudes. Rub this with a hot metal object to melt the plastic and make it fill up the depression. You can use the back of an old spoon for this operation. When heating it up, take care to wrap a cloth round the handle, for this will also get hot. When the plastic is cold, the tee will be fused firmly in place. (If your sports shop only sells wooden golf tees, drill a hole as above and fix the tee in place with wood glue.)

4. Use drawing pins and a magnet
This idea has a strong appeal for children. They seem to see it as some kind of magic! It is really very simple. A steel drawing pin is pushed into each inset piece and a strong round magnet is glued to a handle. (Check that the magnet is the right way round to attract and not repel. Use a firm adhesive like Araldite or Evostick.) Place the magnet on the drawing pin and—Hey Presto!—out comes the inset piece! For children who cannot hold a handle, the magnet can be sewn to a fabric strap with a Velcro fastening. The strap can be worn as a bracelet, or over the child's hand, like a benign knuckle duster! Remember to remove the drawing pins after the play session if there is any chance of them endangering other children.

STABILISING TOYS

Baby Walkers and Dolls' Prams

Some fourwheeled toys can be of a light construction and have their front and back axles fairly close together. These are fine for many children, but those who grasp the handle firmly and lean on it (for support) may tip the toy up. Of course, this situation must be avoided or the child will literally be let down. He could lose confidence and be reluctant to try again. Choose a wheeled toy carefully and think about the size, weight and distance between the wheels. If the toy is a 'hand me down' consider weighting it to make it more stable. Before it ends up in the recycling bin, perhaps an old telephone directory can act as an undermattress. Another idea is to wrap a brick (or two) in cloth. Keep this makeshift cover in place with a few stitches. Position the brick over the front axle of the toy.

A Quick Fix for Light Toys and Paper

- A loop of masking tape. Wind this round your fingers, sticky side out, and overlap the end. Withdraw your fingers, and press the loop flat. You can now use it to stick paper to paper or card.
- Double-sided Sellotape.
- Commercial fixers like Blu-tack, bulldog clips and clothes pegs.

More Durable Fixers for Larger and Heavier Items

- Plastic suckers.
- G cramps.
- A covered brick or therapy bag.
- Dycem mat. This non-slip plastic material is used at sea as a covering for trays. Items carried on the tray will not slide about as the ship rolls. It is also used by disabled adults to steady a mixing bowl, etc. Dycem is available from some of the addresses on p. 7 and can be ordered from the Dispensary at Boots the Chemists.

MAKING TABLE TOP GAMES PLAYABLE

For children who can point with one finger, but who cannot manage to move a counter around a board game, try substituting a Smartie lid. This has a lip which fits a finger tip and makes it easier to slide around the board.

For those who can pinch or have tripod grip, try making this doll on a button. It stands on top of the board. Being three-dimensional, it is easier for some children to control than a flat counter.

Doll on a Button

Quick

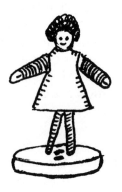

Materials
- A large coat button with a rim.
- Two pipe cleaners.
- Flesh-coloured wool for binding arms and legs (optional).
- Wool for the hair.
- Scrap of old tights and a little polyester filling for the face.
- Embroidery or sewing cotton for the features.
- Scraps of fabric for the clothes (felt is ideal).

Method
Hold the button, rim downwards. To make the legs and body, take one of the pipe cleaners and poke it down through one hole and up through another. Make the legs the same length and pull them up firmly, so that the centre of the pipe cleaner lies close to the underside of the button. Stand the button on the table to check that it lies flat. (If the rim is not thick enough, the pipe cleaner will protrude and the button will rock about. Find another button with a thicker rim!) The finished character must not be top heavy, so keep the legs short, and twist the pipe cleaner about three times in a suitable place to make the body. Leave the ends free for the moment. Take the second pipe cleaner. Hold the ends side by side. Place your little finger in the centre to form a loop for the head. Twist the pipe cleaner about twice to make the neck. Splay out the ends to form the arms. Attach the body to the head and arms by hooking the body ends over the shoulders—like braces. Twist the surplus round the body. Now to finish the arms. Decide on their length in proportion to the body and bend the surplus pipe cleaner ends back towards the neck. Give each arm a twist or two to make it firmer, and to make sure the wire end of the pipe cleaner is safely tucked in.

Now the basic skeleton is finished. All it needs is some character. Pad out the face with the scrap of polyester fibre and cover it with a double layer of tights material. Tie firmly round the neck with cotton and trim off surplus material. Indicate the features with sewing cotton. Make some wool hair with long and short stitches or French knots. To make a good job, bind the arms and legs with flesh-coloured wool (optional if you are making a character wearing long sleeves and trousers!)

Note
These little figures, suitably dressed as a family or as a Police Officer or a Lollipop Lady, etc. come in handy in other situations, such as adding life to a doll's house or a road layout.

Card Games

Cardholders are commercially available for disabled adults. Usually all that children need is a large scrubbing brush! The cards can be firmly supported by the bristles. Alternatively, a few parallel, deep and angled saw cuts in a block of wood can foot the bill.

Highlighting hands

The purpose of this book is to consider ways of helping children who, for whatever reason, need practice in using their hands so that they may function as fully as possible. The first stage in this process may well be highlighting hands—helping a baby or toddler to look at his hands and *realise they are there*!

Left to his own devices a child with a less able hand will tend to ignore it and, very sensibly from the short term point of view, always use the other. With coaxing and by thinking up ways of involving the 'lazy hand' in play, you will stand a much better chance of helping to increase its efficiency.

Here are some well tried *instant* ideas for drawing attention to hands:

SOME WAYS OF DRAWING ATTENTION TO HANDS

- Draw on the child's hands—both of them. (Use non-toxic, water soluble felt tip pens or face paints. The children I have in mind are unlikely to suck their hands or fingers, but you can't be too careful!)
- Paint nails in vivid colours.
- Make a little finger puppet by using an adhesive label. Draw a face on the label, cut it out and stick it to the child's finger.
- Did you ever play 'Cat's Cradle' when you were a child? Those complicated manoeuvres are way beyond the skills of many of the the children in mind, but with your help they can share the pleasant feel of the string (or thick wool) twining between their fingers. In the days when knitting wool came in a skein, I remember watching a therapist help a child trail her fingers through the strands. Remember to tidy away the string when you have finished, just in case it should find its way down the throat of some small child or animal.
- If you have a helium balloon, shorten the string by making a loop on the end. Slip the child's hand through the loop. When she moves her hand, the balloon will move too. A simple lesson in 'cause and effect'!
- Wrist bells serve the same purpose. These can be bought, but are so easy to make, and, of course, this works out cheaper. Just use a pony tail band or a sweat band, according to the size you need, and firmly sew on some bells (from the pet shop).
- Sew metal buttons to the fingers of gloves or to the tips of mitts. Make sure the child has a satisfactory sounding board for her fingers to tap—such as a biscuit tin or a Formica-topped table. This idea has been used for a long time and can often be successful in persuading children to move their fingers. I adapted it once for a rather special need. A physiotherapist friend was working with a little girl who had severely burnt her hand. When her medical treatment was finished, it was necessary to make her hand more flexible. She found it uncomfortable to open and close her hand or to make her fingers touch her

thumb. Using the button idea, I stitched some metal buttons to the hands of a glove puppet. The little girl was happy to manipulate the puppet to 'play the cymbals' in time to a jolly tune on the tape recorder—so that part of the physiotherapy session was happily achieved.

● Long strips of Lammetter (used to decorate Christmas trees) or lengths of thin spaghetti ribbon can also be stitched to the finger ends of gloves. The desire to flick these colourful strips about can be a sure way of encouraging a child to wear the gloves and wiggle her fingers inside!

Zebra Mitts

Long-lasting

I made a trial pair of these for a baby girl with poor sight. Her hands were probably beyond her range of vision and she never played with her fingers as babies usually do. The mitts were made in black and white stripes, zebra fashion. When she brought her hands closer to her eyes, the high contrast in colours would have the best chance of attracting her attention. I was also aiming at a tactile experience for her. If you have ever worn fingerless gloves, you will have noticed how strange they feel when you first put them on, and how extra sensitive your exposed fingers seem to be. While I had the wool handy, I made another pair, just in case it might come in useful sometime . . .

One day Michael, a toddler with hemiplegia, joined the toy library. His Mum said that his right hand was very efficient, but he totally ignored his left. We remembered the Zebra Mitts lurking in the 'oddments box' at the top of the cupboard. Perhaps now was their big moment. We showed the Zebra Mitts to our new little member and tried on a pair. Michael's first reaction was to rip them off! We felt encouraged—at least he was noticing his left hand. We tried again. This time the mitts stayed on for longer, and he patted his left hand with his right. We felt we might be on to something! The Zebra Mitts went home in the toy bag and were used by Michael's therapist in his play sessions. When she reported favourably and asked for several more pairs in different sizes, I knew she would find these useful in highlighting other children's hands.

30

Here is the pattern for Zebra Mitts to fit an average two-year-old. They are knitted in 4ply wool, using size 3 (11) knitting needles. Both hands are the same. To enlarge the pattern, just add a few more stitches and make the stripes a little wider.

There are two styles. The first is only a strip of plain knitting worked in alternate black and white stripes. The second is a little more complicated as it has a gusset for the thumb, and the cuff fits more snugly round the wrist. It is more comfortable to wear, and less easy for the child to pull off!

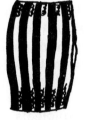

Style 1

Style 1
Cast on 24 stitches in black. Knit 4 rows.
Join in the white wool and K 4 rows.
Repeat these rows three more times. You have now made 4 white stripes—one for each finger.
K 8 rows in black—to wrap round the little finger edge of the hand.
Continue with four more white stripes alternating with black. Cast off (in black).
Wrap your strip of knitting round the child's hand to see where his thumb sticks out.
Stitch the black edges together, remembering to leave a gap for the thumb!
Knit a second mitt the same way.

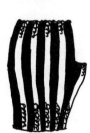

Style 2

Style 2
Starting at the little finger side of the hand, cast on 24 stitches in black.
Knit 2 rows.
Row 3. K 16, turn.
Row 4. Slip the first stitch, then K back across the next 15 stitches. (This part of the mitt, which covers the hand, is wider than the 8 remaining stitches, which fit snugly round the wrist.)
Join in the white wool.
Rows 5 and 6. Knit across all the row.
Rows 7 and 8. As rows 3 and 4.

Repeat rows 5–8 in black, and then in white . . . and so on until you have made four white stripes (one for each finger).

For the thumb gusset (Knitted in black)
Rows 1–3. Knit.
Row 4 (starting at the wrist edge). Slip 1, K 17, turn
Rows 5 and 6. Slip 1, K 9, turn.
Rows 7 and 8. Slip 1, K 7, turn.
Rows 9 and 10. Slip 1, K 5, turn.
Rows 11 and 12. As rows 7 and 8.
Row 13. Slip 1, K 9, turn.
Row 14. Slip 1, K 17 (to edge of cuff.)
Row 15. K 24.
K four more white stripes, alternating and finishing with black. (Keep the cuff stripes narrow as before.) Join up the side seam.
Repeat the pattern for the second mitt.

Hand Prints

Perhaps one of the best ways of focussing on hands is to have a session of hand printing. The child must press his flat hand in a tray (or plate) of paint (*see below*), and then make its imprint on a sheet of paper. For the enthusiastic, a large sheet can be covered with such prints and then used as special wrapping paper. A less messy way of producing hand prints is for the child to rest his flat hand on a sheet of coloured paper. Then comes the best bit for him! YOU draw round his hand

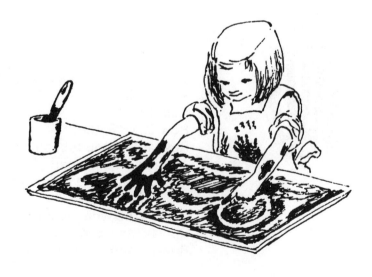

with a pencil and HE experiences a delicious tingle as the pencil trails its way in between his fingers. (Try it!) The resulting shape can be cut out and used in various ways.

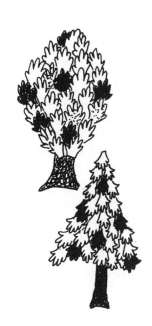

1. *At Linden Bennet School*, each child in the class makes several sets of hand prints and a pair of foot prints. These are cut out and arranged on a large sheet of paper as giant flowers. The foot prints, together with a photograph of the child, form the centre of the flower and the hand prints are arranged around it to make the petals.

2. *At Dysart School*, the teacher draws the outline of a large bird on cheap paper. The outline is filled in with overlapping hand prints, all pointing towards the tail. Arranged this way, they make convincing feathers!

3. *At other schools*, cut out hand prints are used as leaves and, combined together, they make very artistic trees. In Autumn the hand prints are made in red, yellow, brown and orange, to represent the seasonal colours. On the tree, the fingers point upwards. In December there is a demand for more hand prints—dark green this time. These can be mounted with the fingers pointing downwards to represent a Christmas tree.

4. *Single hand prints*, made on card or stiff paper can turn into stick puppets. Turn the hand print this way and that to see what it reminds you of. Perhaps, by rounding off the wrist end, an exotic bird with fantastic tail feathers will come to mind, or a rare tropical fish. You might even use two hand prints, trim off a finger or two, combine them together and

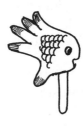 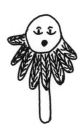

make an octopus. Colour them appropriately, and add any extras, like an eye or a fin. Glue a lolly stick to the back, and you have made a truly unusual stick puppet!

Thick paint for handprints or fingerpainting

It is wise to indulge in this wonderful 'mucky play' in the garden or just before bath time! As a further development, a finger tip or a thumb can be used to make oval shapes for patterns or borders. Print a large shape with the thumb, top it with a smaller shape made by the little finger. With a felt pen, add eyes, ears, whiskers and a tail and you have a cat! These shapes can also convert into an owl, or even the head and body of a person. Turn the shapes on their side, add an eye, a beak, spindly legs and tiny claws, and you have a baby chick!

The first stage in finger painting is usually to give the child two colours, e.g. yellow and blue. Let him experiment and find out for himself, or show him how to mix the colours together to make green. Then he can make paths or patterns in the paint. When that palls, perhaps try 'combing'. For this activity a card 'comb' is dragged across the paint, leaving a trail of parallel stripes. The card needs to be thick or it soons becomes soggy with the paint. Cut uneven V-shaped pieces from one edge. The card left between them will make the stripes. If a child moves the comb through the paint from side to side several times, then from top to bottom, he will have made a plaid pattern. To make another interesting shape try dragging the comb over the paint step fashion—along, then down.

Recipe One

- Flour or cornflour—for use with one child about a cupful should be sufficient.
- A little powder paint.
- Water to mix.

Mix the flour and paint together and gradually add the water, squashing out the lumps, until the mixture is the consistency of thick cream. A pool of cornflour mixture on a Formica-topped table has a strange amoeba-like way of changing its shape. Push it into a pinnacle, and it will subside into a pancake. Press against one edge and it will bulge out somewhere else. Children find this fascinating!

Recipe Two

- About a cup of soapflakes (*not* powdered detergent).
- A little water.
- A little powder paint.

Put the soapflakes and a small amount of powder paint in a bowl. Add a little water and beat to a smooth paste. I am told this recipe can be used to fingerpaint patterns or pictures on the side of the bath!

Rhymes for finger play

Nursery rhymes and jingles have delighted children through the generations. Perhaps the best ones for tiny children are those which we invent on the spot, maybe using the child's name and following it with simple actions, e.g. JENN i FER CLAPS her HANDS, clapping on the syllables or words in capital letters, adding a simple tune and repeating it over and over like a chant! If such spontaneous creativity is not for you, here are some traditional finger plays to fall back on:

Pat-a-Cake

Pat-a-cake, pat-a-cake, baker's man,
Bake me a cake as fast as you can.
(*Hold the child's hands in yours and clap them together in time to the rhythm of the words.*)
Pat it and prick it and mark it with 'B'
(*Guide the child to poke one hand with a finger from the other, then trace the lettershape.*)
And put it in the oven for Baby and me.
(*Wrap your hands round the child's and make a shaking hands movement in time to the words.*)

Of course, this rhyme can be personalised and the child's initial and name used instead of 'B' and 'Baby'.

FINGERS AND THUMBS

Round and Round the Garden

Here is another perennial favourite:

Round and round the garden, like a teddy bear,
(*Trail your finger round the child's palm with a circular movement.*)
One step, two step, tickle me under there!
(*Walk your fingers up the child's arm and tickle in a different place every time.*)

We'll All Clap Hands Together

This jingle is a good one for family or group play:

We'll all clap hands together,
We'll all clap hands together,
We'll all clap hands together,
As children like to do.

Other verses might be 'We wiggle our fingers together' ... etc. or 'We open and close together' ... etc. Invent the words to suit your needs.

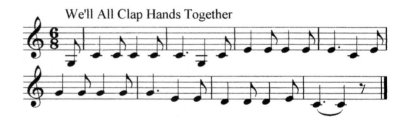

We'll All Clap Hands Together

Clap, Clap Hands, One, Two, Three

Clap, clap hands, one, two, three
(*Clap in time to the rhythm of the words.*)
Put your hands on your knees
(*Do the action.*)
Lift them high to touch the sky
(*Do the action.*)
Clap, clap hands, and away they fly
(*Suit the action to the words.*)

Here is a Tree with Leaves so Green

Here is a tree with leaves so green
(*Hold your hands with the fingers pointing upwards to represent the branches.*)
Here are the apples that hang between
(*Make hands into fists.*)

36

When the wind blows the apples fall
(*Flutter fingers.*)
Here is a basket to gather them all
(*Interlace fingers to form the basket.*)

Tommy Thumb Where are You?

In this rhyme the digits on one hand appear to talk to the matching ones on the other. Say the thumb and fingers on the left hand ask the questions, make a fist of the right hand and pop the thumb and fingers out as the questions are asked.

Q. Tommy Thumb, Tommy Thumb, where are you?
(*Waggle thumb as if it was talking.*)
A. Here I am, here I am. How do you do?
(*Waggle other thumb as if replying.*)

Q. Peter Pointer, Peter Pointer, where are you?
(*First finger waggles.*)
A. Here I am, Here I am. How do you do?

Q. Middle Man, Middle Man, where are you?
(*Action and reply as before.*)

Q. Ruby Ring, Ruby Ring, where are you?
(*Ring—third—finger in action.*)

Q. Baby Small, Baby Small, where are you?
(*Fourth finger . . .*)

Make a fist of right hand again before this final verse.

Q. Fingers all, Fingers all, where are you?
A. Here we are, here we are. How do you do?
(*Open hand rapidly.*)

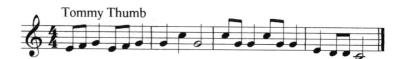

Tommy Thumb

Toys for putting on hands

FINGER PUPPETS

These delightful little toys do not appear in museums, and I wonder if they have evolved from the strips of stamp paper countless mothers—including mine—stuck to the fingernails of their children's index fingers for the fun of playing 'Two Little Dicky Birds' (Peter and Paul) ... who fly away and then come back again. Nowadays finger puppets, usually made in felt, are found in many toy and craft shops. When Christmas draws near and we are all eager for little novelties and quickly-made toys, patterns appear in magazines. Made to represent characters in a nursery rhyme or fairy story, they make splendid small presents. They are also great for journeys or as a little reward or consolation in a crisis. Any Mum, Auntie or Grandmother who makes a few to keep by for an emergency will bless the day she had such forethought! We notice the child appeal that finger puppets have when it is time for the music session at the toy library. Mums, dads and children gather round the piano in a semicircle to join in the finger plays and action songs. It is noticeable that the ones which include finger puppets hold the children's interest best. Their hand movements are larger and freer, and even the shy ones will join in. For children with hand function problems, finger puppets may play a special part. They certainly focus attention on hands, and they can help a child to move one finger in isolation from the others.

At first, the best way of using finger puppets is for you to wear a pair on your index fingers, while your child has a smaller pair on hers. Now you are all set to act out the 'Two Little Dicky Birds' and other rhymes described below. Older children may be able to make more sophisticated characters and act out stories.

How to make finger puppets

Instant

To make a finger puppet in a jiffy, simply draw a little face on the front of a finger, yours or a child's, and wrap a handkerchief or tissue round it. It is immediately dressed in a hood and cloak! Keep this rudimentary clothing in place with a rubber band.

Very Quick

If you have an old pair of fabric gloves, cut off the best fingers and embellish them as suits your fancy, or as play dictates. Put your finger inside the potential puppet. This makes it easier to work on. Draw the eyes and mouth with felt pens or, if these will not show up well, indicate them with a few stitches. Stick on some wool or fur fabric 'hair' (PVA adhesive). Add some felt clothes, stitched or stuck, or use layers of lampshade trimming for a 1920s dress!

Quick

Now we come to the finger puppet for knitters to make. The basic pattern is worked in stocking stitch. It can be made from odd scraps of wool, and the knitting part can

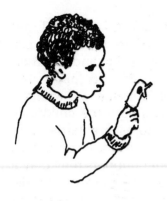

be completed in less than twenty minutes! This makes it an excellent project for children who are just learning to knit, because the puppet is finished before boredom sets in. If the body is knitted in stripes, it will appear to grow even more quickly.

Here is the basic pattern for an adult's finger. I suggest you follow it and try it for size. Then subtract a few stitches and knit a few less rows to make one to fit a child. Allowing for the head and neck, the finished puppet's body should just cover the second joint of the index finger. (If it is too short and wide, it is likely to fall off, if too long and narrow, it is a struggle to fit it on.)

Method
Use Double Knitting (DK) wool and size 3¾ (9) or 3¼ (10) needles. (With thinner wool use finer needles and cast on a few more stitches.)
Cast on 14 sts.
Knit two rows plain.
Knit 14 rows stocking stitch for the body. (One row plain, one row purl.)
Knit 10 rows stocking stitch for the head. (This will be a different colour if you are making a person.)
Break off a long length of wool and thread it through the stitches on the needle. Draw the wool up tightly to gather the stitches together for the top of the head. Join the sides of your knitting together so that the puppet now looks like the finger of a glove.

Make the head by pushing a small ball of polyester fibre into the tip. Bind with wool, just below the head. This will keep the filling in place and make a neck.

Now all your puppet needs is some individuality. The easiest character to make is a little bird. Just give your puppet two black French knot eyes, and sew on a diamond-shaped felt beak in a contrasting colour.

Some ways of using this pattern

Two Little Dicky Birds

Knit another bird for yourself and a smaller pair for your child and you are ready to play 'Two Little Dicky Birds'. Here is the rhyme and the actions that go with it:

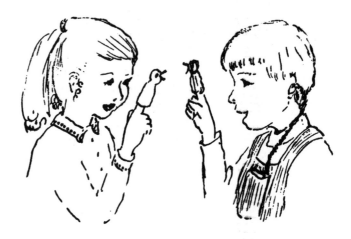

Two little dicky birds sitting on a wall,
(*Let puppets peep over the back of a chair or edge of the table.*)
One named Peter,
(*Hold him up high*)
The other named Paul.
(*Hold him up too*)
Fly away Peter,
(*Hide him behind your back*)
Fly away Paul,
(*Hide him too*)
Come back Peter,
(*Bring him out from behind your back*)
Come back Paul.
(*Bring him out too*)

Two Grand Ladies

For the 'Two Grand Ladies', knit two puppets, changing to a flesh colour after the 14 rows stocking stitch. Make the ladies as grand as possible by adding wool hair, a felt hat with a feather in it, a satin cloak embellished with sequins . . . let your imagination run riot!

This is their rhyme:

Two grand ladies met in the lane,
(*Have the puppets on your index fingers, hold them apart and gradually bring them together*)
Bowed most politely, bowed once again.
(*Make your fingers match the words and bow to each other*)

41

'How do you do?'
(*One finger bows*)
'How do you do?'
(*The other bows*)
And 'How do you do?' again.
(*Both bow*)

Five Little Ducks

Knit the basic pattern five times in yellow, add black eyes and orange bills, and you have the five little ducks that went swimming. Make the Mother Duck as a snapper, using the pattern suggested on p. 110. Here is the rhyme and tune for them:

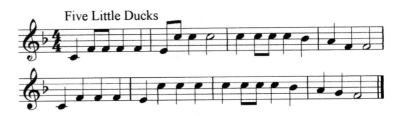

Five Little Ducks

Five little ducks went swimming one day,
Over the pond and far away.
(*Wear a duck on all the fingers of one hand and make them 'swim' across the pond*)
Mother Duck said 'Quack, quack, quack',
(*Use snapper puppet with the other hand, in time to the words*)
And *four* little ducks came swimming back.
(*Remove one puppet or bend your finger down*)

Four little ducks went swimming one day, etc.

Repeat until . . .
No little ducks came swimming back.

Last verse . . .
Mother Duck went swimming one day,
Over the pond and far away.
Mother Duck said 'Quack, quack, quack',
And *five* little ducks came swimming back

It is possible that you have now become addicted to knitting finger puppets! I guess you will think of many more characters to make. Here are two suggestions to start you off:

A Snowman

Knit the puppet in white, add a black felt hat, features and a brightly coloured scarf.

A Guardsman

Start to knit in black for his trousers, change to red for his tunic, give him a pink face and top him with a black busby. Give him features and a wool chin strap. Add gold French knot buttons to his tunic and a felt belt.

Finger Puppets with Arms

Quick

These finger puppets take a little longer to make than the basic pattern above, but the result is a more convincing person with greater potential for imaginative play. If the puppet is knitted for an individual child, it can be made to represent a member of the family by giving it identifying characteristics—perhaps glasses for grandma, a bald head for grandpa, and so on.

Materials
Needles and scraps of wool, including a flesh colour, as for the finger puppets above.

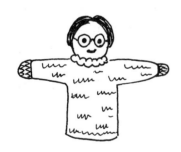

Method
The front and back are identical. They are knitted separately, then partly stitched together at the head and shoulders so that the hands can be added. Finally, the under arms and side seams are joined together.
Here is the pattern. Knit it twice.

Cast on 8 st.
K 2 rows plain. K 12 rows stocking stitch.

The Arms. Cast on 4 st. K into the back of the first 5 st., then K to the end of the row.
Cast on 4 st. P into the back of the first 5, then P to the end of the row. (16 st.)
K 1 row.
P 1 row.
Cast off 6 st. (to make the shoulders). K to the end of the row.
Cast off 6 st. P to end of the row. (4 st.)

The Head. Break off the body colour and tie in the flesh colour.

K into the front and back of the first st., K 2. K into the front and back of the last st. (6 st.)

P 1 row.

Increase 1 st. at the beginning and end of the next row. (8 st.)

P 1 row.

Work 4 rows stocking stitch.

K 2 tog. at both ends of the next row. (6 st.)

P 1 row.

K 2 tog. at both ends of the next row. Break off wool and thread through the remaining 4 st. Do not cut it off. It is needed for sewing the sides of the head together.

Knit the other half of the puppet the same way.

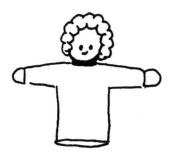

With right sides together, join the front and back from the top of the head to the end of the arms. (Use the matching wool left over from drawing up the head stitches.)

Now add the *hands.* Using flesh colour, pick up nine stitches across the end of one sleeve. K 4 rows of stocking stitch. Break off wool. Thread through the stitches, draw up and stitch together the sides of the hand. Repeat the process for the other hand.

Complete the joining up.

Stuff the head with a small ball of polyester fibre and tie round the neck.

Bring your puppet to life by adding features, hair, and extra adornments—buttons made from French knots, a lace collar, or perhaps a hat?

The standard puppet lends itself to variations. The body can be knitted in two colours to represent jeans and a jersey, fabric clothes can be added—even 'props' like a tiny duster can be stitched to one hand, or a pom-pom ball tucked under a child puppet's arm. To make a baby, simply reduce the pattern by casting on less stitches (say 6) and working fewer rows.

GLOVE PUPPETS

Bought glove puppets are often too large and heavy for small hands, but it is easy for anyone handy with a needle to make one the right size.

First cut out a paper pattern. Place the child's hand on a piece of paper with the fingers and thumb in the positions they will adopt when working the puppet. Most children like to use their thumb for one arm, their index finger for the neck and their middle finger for the other arm. The ring and little fingers are tucked into the palm. A few children prefer to use two fingers to work the head and two fingers for the arm not filled with the thumb. Draw round the child's hand in his chosen position, making a very generous seam allowance. Cut out the puppet in double material and tack round the seams. Try it for size before stitching properly, then decorate according to character. A slit up the back of the puppet's dress can make it much easier for some children to put their fingers in the right places.

See also
Glove puppet with buttons on hands (p. 29).

A Glove Puppet Made From a Sock

Instant or Quick

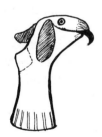

Some readers may remember the TV puppeteer Sharri Lewis and her endearing socklike glove puppet 'Lambchop'. This type of puppet is very easy to make and in its simplest form is definitely *instant*! Just put the sock over your hand, and extend your fingers and thumb so that they are in opposition. Poke the tip of the toe of the sock between your fingers and thumb to make a small pocket which represents the mouth. Already you can move your fingers and thumb apart and together to make the sock appear to talk. In this crude state the sock puppet will probably soon lose its 'mouth'! Withdraw your hand and make a few stitches at the sides of the mouth to keep the pocket (formed by the tucked-in toe) folded in. Use felt to add floppy ears, and a tongue. Button eyes can look effective. With wool, sew nostrils, eyebrows (and whiskers?). For children to use, this puppet must have all its characteristic decorations sewn on very securely. I prefer to use a sock with a long leg, which will partly cover my arm. For some children it may be better to choose a short sock, which will fit more easily over their hand.

Holding on

Offer a new-born baby your finger to hold and you will notice the almost vice-like grip in his tiny fingers. This ability to clutch is one of the hand-function skills most of us are born with. It is certainly a very useful one. For some children this simple action may not be automatic and they must learn to close their fingers round an object. Of course, if the reason for performing this action is sufficiently attractive, the child is more likely to be motivated to persist. This is where a carefully chosen toy can come to the rescue. Some children favour certain textures, and a toy with that covering may have an appeal. (You find this out by trial and error!) Most seem to go for one that makes a noise and this is where the traditional rattle plays its part. The usual baby rattle may not be appropriate for a child who finds it difficult to grasp. Here are some suggestions for some (mostly home-made) rattles of an unusual shape. Perhaps one among this collection will fill the bill.

A Spherical Rattle

Instant

If you are looking for a round rattle that will fit neatly in the palm of a child's hand and the toy shop cannot oblige, try the pet shop! Here you will find a cat ball with a bell inside. It is made in brightly-coloured plastic, and has holes here and there—like a golf practice ball.

Quick

If you need a larger round rattle and one that is soft to the touch, use one of the ball patterns in the section on throwing and catching (p. 93). Put your own noisemaker in the middle. This might be a film carton containing a couple of bells or some fishgrit (*see* p. 6). The stuffing in the ball will tend to dampen the sound, so punch a few holes in the film carton for a better effect.

A Rattle from a Fruit Squash Bottle

Instant

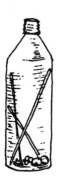

This rattle is ideal for a child who has just learnt to sit up, or who is lying over a wedge to play. It is a good size for grasping, and its light weight and transparency give it child appeal. A smaller mineral water bottle may fit some hands better. Its owner is likely to spend ages just shaking the bottle, watching the contents bob about inside and trying to make the loudest possible noise.

First wash the bottle thoroughly, then make sure it is really dry. If any moisture remains inside, it will form condensation, which will obscure the contents, and they may stick together and not rattle properly. Practically any filling that will go through the neck may be used but, in the interests of safety, it is best to stick to edible items like spaghetti, rice, lentils, etc. If you are *certain* the child will not manage to undo the lid, a few brightly-coloured buttons and some scraps of foil paper will look more attractive, and possibly make a louder noise. Once the contents are inside, the lid must be fixed on securely with polystyrene cement (e.g. U-Hu). Make sure this is set before offering the rattle to the child.

A Strong Rattle from a Washing-up Liquid Bottle

Instant or Quick (if painted)

This rattle is much more robust than the one above, and will stand a heavier filling. This could be a useful point if the rattle is to be used by a child with flaccid hands. The weight might be adjusted to suit her strength, and possibly improve her muscular tone. (I believe in Sweden some of the play dolls used in therapy are weighted with different amounts of sand.)

For safety reasons, fix the stopper in place with polystyrene cement, and cut off the small plastic plug and the loop which attaches it to the stopper. The bottle will now have a hole in the top. This will add to its attraction, for it can also be used as a puffer.

The outside of the bottle can be made more decorative by scrubbing off the printing with wire wool, then decorating it with a pattern painted with Humbrol enamel. This paint is quite safe for children, dries quickly, does an excellent cover-up job, and will not crack when the bottle is squeezed.

Special Rattles for Frail Children and those with Small Hands

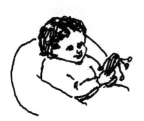

The need here is usually for extra small and light rattles.

- One teacher uses a Tic-Tac sweet container, puts in a few grains of rice and seals down the lid by binding it to the container with plastic tape.
- An empty film carton can soon be transformed into a small cylindrical rattle. A parent who attends the toy library showed me one she had made for her little daughter. She put a bell inside the carton, (it could have been fish grit or rice) replaced the lid, and covered the whole thing with a crochet cover worked in fine, brightly-coloured wools. The cover made the rattle visually attractive, less slippery to hold, and made certain the lid could not come off. (A few holes punched in the carton made the bell sound louder.)
- A therapist asked me to make a very slender rattle for a small baby. He had been born with his thumbs clenched in the palms of his hands. She hoped that placing a thin rattle under his thumbs for short periods might gradually loosen the tightness of his grip. She suggested making the shank of the rattle about the diameter of a felt pen.

  From then on I was on my own! I searched for a suitable shank and found a narrow fibre pen. I vandalised it and removed its messy inside. I cut it down to what I considered to be the right size to fit a tiny palm and set about introducing a noise-making element. I threaded some thin round hat elastic through the loop on a bell, put the ends of the elastic together and threaded them through the fibrepen shank. Now the rattle had a bell on one end. It was easy to thread a single piece of elastic through another bell, pull the elastic really tight, and tie a knot. I trimmed off most of the surplus elastic and slid the bells along their elastic loop until the knot was hidden inside the shank. With a bell fixed at both ends the rattle now looked just like a miniature dumb-bell.

I felt its appearance would be improved by a covering of fabric and, if the baby should wave his new rattle about excitedly, the soft exterior would prevent him from scratching himself. I cut a circle of fabric (it happened to be lycra) large enough to cover a bell. I stretched it over the top of the bell and bound it tightly to the shank with double cotton. It was too bulky, so it was unwrapped, and wedge-shaped pieces were cut from the circumference of the circle. Now it fitted round the shank more snugly. I repeated the process with the other bell, then wound a short strip of fabric round the shank to cover all that binding. The strip was kept in place with a row of stitches down the length of the shank. Result ... one tiny, easily grasped rattle!

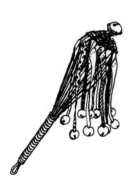

● An unusual twirly rattle—highly acclaimed by all the children to whom I have given one—has been invented by Alison Wisbeach. Its skeleton is a small metal egg whisk. Short lengths of ribbon, each a different bright colour, have a bell stitched to one end. The other ends are attached to the whisk by wrapping them round alternate loops of wire and stitching them in place. If left to their own devices, the ribbons tend to slip to the bottom of the whisk and tangle together. This can be avoided by making a sort of spider's web to fill in the bottom. In wool, backstitch over each loop of wire in turn. Press the strands of wool together, and keep them in place with a few stitches between the loops of wire—like the spokes of an umbrella. An extra bell added to the centre of this web gives the rattle a more finished look and adds to its noisemaking potential.

Rattles for older children

A Jumbo Shaker

Quick

Rosemary Hemmett,
Toy Librarian

Have you ever searched in vain for a *really* large rattle? Here is one that is suitable for an older child, who still needs this type of toy. In this case 'baby' rattles are too small and fragile, and neither attractive nor appropriate. Rosemary uses a tough plastic salad shaker that looks like two colanders joined together by a hinge. Normally, freshly washed lettuce is placed inside and rapidly shaken to remove all the surplus water. Replace the lettuce with ping-pong balls or, better still, cat balls (each with a bell inside) from the pet shop. Tie the two halves of the salad shaker together at intervals round the edge and bind the handles together. You now have a large, strong rattle that can be carried about or hung up to be biffed.

A Slither Box

Quick

This rattle makes an intriguing sound. It can be used to imitate the noise of footsteps on gravel or, tilted more slowly, it can make you think of waves breaking on a stony beach. It contains fish grit (used in aquaria). The feeling of the weight being transferred from one hand to the other as the grit slides about inside the box seems to fascinate children. When one boy first held it, he spent ages slowly turning it over and over in an attempt to make a continuous sound. Its unusual shape and noise-making potential makes it attractive to older children, who have thoroughly explored the possibilities of other percussion instruments. Be generous with the papier mâché layers that cover it, and it will be very strong.

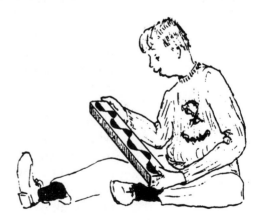

Method
You will need to find a large, flat cardboard box—like the one in the illustration—the longer the better if you want to use it to encourage a child to use a 'lazy' hand. Put in a few spoonfuls of fish grit or, for a softer sound, use rice, dried peas, etc.—experiment! Next, using flour and water paste (p. 5) or PVA adhesive, watered down for economy, first cover the box with a layer of strips of torn newspaper, then go all over it again with a different sort of paper (e.g. computer paper). Repeat this process at least once more, or until the box is really rigid and strong. By using alternate layers of different kinds of paper, it is easier to avoid leaving areas uncovered. Wait for the box to be thoroughly dry. Apply an undercoat of pale emulsion paint. When that is dry, decorate the box with a bold all-over pattern using Humbrol enamel, or water-based paint, and add a final protective cover of two coats of polyurethane varnish.

Now for some more percussion instruments.

Bell Shakers with an Easy-grip Handle

Quick

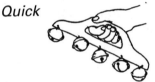

For children who find it difficult to grasp, it can be worthwhile making bell shakers from wooden workbag handles, obtainable from a craft shop or, maybe, a car boot sale! Along the bottom edge of the handles (where the bag is usually attached), drill a few holes far enough apart for the bells to hang independently of each other.

A Scraper

Instant or Quick

In its instant form, the perfect scraper is an old-fashioned washboard possibly dug out from the attic. Some readers may remember that back in the 1950s a washboard formed the rhythm section of a skiffle group. Younger readers will have no idea what I am talking about! A washboard came into its own on wash days. It was a sheet of corrugated metal mounted on a wooden frame. It stood in the washtub and our grandmothers would drape a grubby article of clothing over it and attack it with a bar of Sunlight soap and a scrubbing brush. If only a washboard was on sale now, we could show a child how to rub a drum stick across the ridges to make an unusual and captivating sound.

Better still, dispense with the stick, and put thimbles on his fingers. This way he would have a close affinity with the sound produced, and would experience a delicious tingling sensation in his fingertips.

If you like the washboard idea, try making one from some ridged material. A trip to the DIY store could produce fluted pelmet board, ridged doorstep protector or some other unlikely material for a toy! Beware of sharp edges which, of course, must be covered. One parent mounted some metal ridges with narrow corrugations, on wood. He surrounded the edges with beading, like a picture frame. The result was a heavy, but very strong and safe percussion instrument, which delighted his son and made him the envy of all his friends.

Drums

The drumstick used to stroke the washboard may remind you of that perennial toy, the 'kitchen drum'. All you need for this is a stout upturned saucepan and a wooden spoon (or two). Presented to a child at the right age and stage, and the appeal of this 'toy' is audibly evident!

I have tried to make a drum, but so far have not been successful. It is so difficult to keep the head in place and really taut. Maybe once the saucepan drum is outgrown, there is nothing for it but to visit the toy shop.

Perhaps you have noticed a small child looking longingly at a drum but, because of the shape of his hand, he is unable to grasp or control the stick. Jason had this problem. His fingers were curled and stiff. After some thought we arranged for him to have his big moment at the weekly toy library music session. A stout rubber band was stretched over the head of a drum. By hooking his fingers under the band, Jason could stretch it, then slip his fingers out to make it twang against the drum head. He used this skill to good purpose when it came to singing 'Pop goes the Weasel'. We all sang the words so far, then waited for Jason to give his dramatic 'pop' before finishing off the verse.

Fiddle toys

Whatever our age, it seems there are times when we all love to 'fiddle'—running something through our fingers for the sheer pleasure of it. Imagine sitting on the beach, sifting the hot, dry sand through your fingers, or fiddling with an elastic band. I suppose even stroking the cat might be considered a 'fiddle'! Activities like these are relaxing and give us a pleasant tactile experience. For children with hand-function problems, they can be more than that. The act of 'fiddling' is not just a way of passing the time. It can often strengthen fingers and help to make them more supple. Children are normally inveterate fiddlers, and usually find their own favourite objects.

However, some may not be sufficiently mobile to manage this and might welcome a ready-made fiddle toy. Here are some suggestions.

A Serendipity of Fiddle Toys

Almost Instant
(Just allow a little time to collect them all)

Dr Lilli Nielson,
Danish expert on the education of visually impaired children

Lilli Nielson has a magic suitcase full of bits and pieces guaranteed to please any child with a passion for fiddling. With such motivation, lots of finger and hand movements (and tactile experience) are bound to follow. Lift the lid of the suitcase and you will find . . .

- About four strings of beads and buttons, joined together at one end so that they form a tassel.
- Old bed springs with the ends bent in and protected with sticky tape.
- A pliable soap saver with little plastic suckers on the reverse side.
- A bunch of real keys on a strong ring, with a wooden tag to dangle them by.
- An embroidery frame with tracing paper stretched tightly over it, making it like a flat little drum.
- An electric toothbrush holder (without the brush), battery driven. Switch it on and off to experience the pleasant vibration.
- Three long strands of material, loosely plaited together, so that small fingers can wiggle between the strands.
- A bunch of Bendy Straws, taped together at one end, so that the bendy parts at the other can be twisted about in different directions.
- Large buttons on a loop of elastic.
- Plenty of rattles and tins with something in them to shake about.

One can imagine any child saying to itself 'Just let me get at that lot!'

A Chain in a Bottle

Almost instant

Hettie Whitby,
Teacher

This is a simple, but intriguing, fiddle toy—one of the best I have come across. If you are familiar with Winnie-the-Pooh and his friends, you will know the story of Eeyore's birthday present. Pooh and Piglet meant to give him a jar of honey and a balloon, but one got accidentally popped and the other absentmindedly eaten. He ended up with a damp bit of rubbery rag and an empty honey jar. To his infinite satisfaction, Eeyore found that he could put the popped balloon in the honey jar,and take it out again! His friends left him happily repeating this action over and over again. This toy has the same appeal. As Eeyore said: 'It goes in . . . and it comes out'!

The bottle is a discarded plastic one that has a handle moulded into it. In its working life, it probably contained fabric softener. It is a pretty blue and, of course, the handle makes it easy to grasp. The chain can be bought from the local ironmongers (or DIY store). The length needed is about twice the height of the bottle. In theory, the chain should stick to the bottom of the bottle with a blob of Araldite. I must confess mine did not. Perhaps the bottle was damp! But it was a simple matter to *stitch* the chain to the bottom of the bottle by squinting through the neck and poking a long needle, threaded with button thread, in through one side of the bottle, through the end link and out through the other side. I repeated the process several times, in effect binding the chain to the bottom of the bottle. A child can have fun dropping the chain in the bottle and shaking it out again, but for most children it is better to go one step further and tie a ring or a cotton reel to the free end of the chain. This makes it easy to hold and prevents it from totally disappearing inside the bottle. Offer this peculiar toy to a child who has just learnt to sit independently, or to an older one who has a craze for 'fiddle' toys, and you are sure to have a happy and satisfied customer!

TACTILE TOYS

At one stage of my working life, I taught children who had once been sighted, but who had recently become blind as the result of an illness. My task was to try to help them over the initial stages of their loss of sight— to show them how their finger tips (and their ears) could help them to make sense of their new world. Once their confidence was won and they were not afraid to reach out for new experiences, I noticed how 'curious' their fingers became—pinching, stroking and thoroughly exploring the strange toys I made for them. This digital activity might be called 'fiddling for a purpose' for I wanted them to identify articles and textures by touch— and not by sight as had been their habit. The examples of simple tactile toys that follow may also help a child with a hand-function problem to use fingers and thumb to better effect.

Tactile Bags

Quick

These are made like beanbags (p. 92), but the contents are chosen for their variety and tactile appeal. Ideally, the covers should be fairly thin, so that the contents are hidden, but can be easily felt through the fabric. The idea is to put at least two articles in each bag, so that the child can separate them out by wiggling them about inside. As usual, select items suitable for the child or group in mind. For children with sharp teeth, it may be necessary to use tougher material. Be extra fussy about the contents and make sure they will do no harm if eaten (i.e. go for larger items, like a spoon and a tooth brush, or stick to food like rice and pasta). The bags must be made to withstand much pulling, squeezing and pinching, so sew all seams twice and be fussy about closing the gap (where you insert the filling) securely.

Here are some possible fillings to start you thinking.

- A crunched-up potato crisp bag and a ping-pong ball.
- Rice and a few large buttons.
- Two curtain rings and some dried peas.
- Orange pips and a marble.
- A cotton reel and some coins or Lego bricks.

Other possible contents might be ... large beads, bricks (plastic or wood), nylon pan scrubber, large shells, Smartie tops, a squeaky toy, a rattle or everyday objects, like a comb or a key.

Grab Bags

Instant or Quick

These are just an enlarged and tougher version of the tactile bags above. They are intended to be used by children with an iron grip, and are useful for hanging on many of the toy supports suggested in the section on Making Play Possible (p. 11).

For an instant version, use the strong net bags used to package onions, oranges, etc. Partly fill the bag with conkers or acorns in season, or nuts, or shiny crunchy plastic packaging, (from a box of tarts?) and there you are!

For the quick version, you might start off with a small tin. Inside, put bells from a broken toy, or buttons, or a few grains of rice. Glue and/or tape the lid on, and enclose the tin in a bag made from brightly-coloured, very strong material such as upholstery fabric or deck chair canvas.

An Amorphous Beanbag

Quick

Sylvia O'Bryan,
Tutor,
Toymaking Course

As its name suggests, this beanbag is a wholly unconventional shape. This, of course, is part of its attraction. The body of the beanbag is about the size of a dinner plate, but its shape is anything but circular. Look at the picture and you may be reminded of a 'treasure island' with lots of bays and peninsulas, a much more interesting beanbag shape than the conventional square or oblong. Add a bunch of ribbons or a plait or a small toy to the projecting parts of this beanbag and loosely fill it with dried peas (or fish grit if it will need washing).

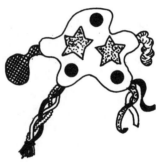

A Manx Feely Cushion

Quick

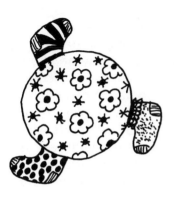

This circular cushion, like the emblem for the Isle of Man, has three legs. It is a convenient way of keeping three fiddle bags together and is specially useful in group situations where small toys tend to get scattered around the room. The legs are just odd, brightly-coloured socks with a tactile or noisemaking object inside.

Materials
- A dinner plate for a template.
- Some interesting fabric such as velvet or fur fabric for the cushion. The back and front could be different.
- Three small socks, toddler size.
- A filling for each sock—noisy or tactile.

Method

Use the dinner plate as a template and cut out two circles of fabric. Take the three socks and put a noisemaker or something tactile in each. Tack across the top of each sock to keep the contents inside. Take one circle of fabric and lay it down, right side up. Take a sock and place its top on the circumference of the circle with the toe pointing towards the centre. Pin it in place. Repeat the process with the other two socks, spacing them at equal intervals apart. Put the other circle of fabric, rightside downwards, on top of the socks. Pin and tack both circles together round the circumference, making sure you have caught in the tops of the socks. Then stitch firmly most of the way round the edge, leaving a gap between two socks for turning and stuffing. Oversew the seam. Turn the cushion right side out. Stuff with polyester filling or crunched-up news-paper or what you will. Close the gap.

A Tactile Junk Box

Instant

Every child should have one! This magical collection of bits and bobs, kept in its own container, such as an ice cream tub or a strong cardboard box, costs nothing and can be the best toy ever. We have all known children who have initially ignored an expensive toy, but spent ages playing with the wrapping paper or the box. A Tactile Junk Box capitalises on this kind of play. It is nothing more than a collection of *safe* rubbish . . . perhaps an egg box with its floppy lid and exciting little indentations, a large piece of bubbly plastic, a short length of thick (unswallowable) metal or plastic chain, some empty cotton reels, the packaging from a box of jam tarts, a carrot or a lemon—the list can go on and on, always subject to the *safety factor* and the age and habits of the child, and possibly his playmates.

The contents of the box can be changed as often as fresh delights occur to you. Its function may be altered as the child grows older, and it need not be restricted to tactile objects. With its contents updated, it can become a 3D box of memories. Perhaps now it will contain shells brought home from a holiday, or souvenirs which are a reminder of a special occasion. Whatever the outcome, such a box can have a healthy influence on any child's incidental learning through play. Textures, colours, shapes, and smells can all have their place within it.

Such diversity can only enrich a child's experience and, as well as giving plenty of practice in handling objects of different sizes and weight, may even help to develop language, observation, and memory! (Can't be bad!)

Exploring with fingers

FEELY BOXES

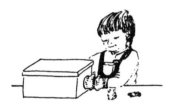

In my youth, the bran tub at the village fête was always surrounded by a group of children, eager to see what they could fish out. Bran tubs with their special smell and texture seem to have been replaced by lucky dips, which are often no more than a bucket full of colour-fully-wrapped little bundles. Less messy no doubt, but the children completely miss out on the mystery and excitement of the old bran tub. Never mind. Feely boxes can help to give some of that feeling of mystery and anticipation as children grope inside and make their choice by touch and not by sight. What a satisfactory way of wiggling your fingers to some purpose! You might choose two toys, show them to the child and let her examine them, put them in the box, and invite her to pull out her favourite one. Or you could put in one toy (unseen by the child) and see if she can guess what it is. At a later stage, familiar objects like a mug or a tooth brush can take the place of a toy. It may be best to choose unthreatening and pleasantly tactile objects at first, though I know one child who has been known to scrabble around happily for ice blocks or even blobs of shaving foam!

An *Instant* Feely Box

Nina Hanson,
Humberside Toy
Libraries

Use a strong cardboard box. One from the Off Licence could be suitable. Put this in an old nylon stretch cushion cover. The elasticated opening will gather nicely round the top, leaving a hole for the children to dip into.

Another Carton Feely Box

Very Quick

Nursery Nurses,
Bedelsford School

If the carton has flaps for a lid, tape them together with parcel tape and turn the box upside down. (Flaps are now at the bottom.) Cut two holes in the new top. These are for the child's arms to reach into the box. On the opposite side where you will sit, cut a door flap so that you can secretly change the items in the box. Now you are ready for action. A child puts her hands through the holes in the top. You lift the flap and maybe pop in a square brick. When this has been successfully identified, change it for a ball or a soft toy. If the feely box is to be used often, it might be worth while covering the sides with wrapping paper (possibly made from hand prints?) or a collage of old Christmas cards. It is best not to decorate the top—pictures here could distract the child from the job in hand, which is wiggling her fingers and thinking about the object she is trying to identify by touch.

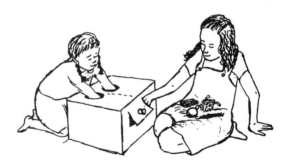

A Smaller Feely Box

Almost Instant

Chris Baker,
Toy Librarian

Use a shoe box. Remove the lid and cut out a rectangle in both ends of the box. One is for the child's hand, the other for yours. Cut a curtain of fabric large enough to cover the child's rectangle and stick it in place along the top of the inside of the opening. Replace the lid and put the box on the table. Now you can put objects in through your hole, while the child tries to find out what is hidden behind the curtain on her side.

Discrimination Bags

Instant

These serve the same purpose as feely boxes, and can be useful for children who are not too keen on reaching into the unknown! All you need is a draw-string bag, such as a shoe bag, and some interesting shapes to put inside. Because the contents are covered by the fabric, they must be identified by touch. If the child's curiosity is sufficiently aroused, his fingers will be eager to squeeze, pinch and turn about the object(s) inside.

Perhaps he will identify his drinking cup, his squeaky toy or his spoon. If he is learning to recognise shapes, here is a good opportunity to reinforce by touch what he is already able to identify by sight. When he thinks he has discovered the hidden contents of his bag, he can open the top and check his guess.

Pulling

This is another of those hand movements we are unconsciously using all the time, gathering articles closer to us, pulling a string to make something happen—even taking the spoon out of the jam needs a pulling movement. Most children add this useful skill to their repertoire without even thinking about it and by the time they can toddle, all sorts of wheeled toys will happily be pulled along behind them. Others may need to be coaxed to wrap their fingers round something and *pull*. For these children, here are some practical suggestions.

Just Pulling

Instant

Christine Cousins,
Educational
Psychologist

1. *Give the child a box of tissues*, preferably the decorative kind usually found on dressing tables. Let her pull the tissues out, one by one, through the hole in the centre of the top. Collect up the tissues for future use or for a game of tug-of-war with big brother!

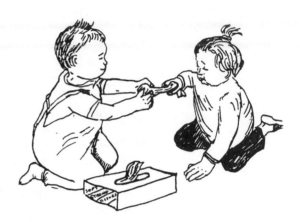

2. *Start off with a polythene ice cream carton* (or similar). Make a hole in the lid. String together many strips of thin material. (Make sure the knots will go through the hole in the lid.) Pile all the material neatly in the container, thread the end through the hole. Put the lid on firmly and invite the child to start pulling. She will be amazed at the seemingly endless string of materials she is producing and will, surely, be motivated to carry on to the bitter end. This toy reminds me of the yards of silk handkerchiefs magicians can produce from the most unlikely places.

PULLING A STRING

The Tumbling Tower

Instant

Roy McConkey,
Vice-President,
National Association
of Toy and Leisure
Libraries

Place a wide piece of ribbon over the edge of the table. Pile a stack of foam bricks on top of the ribbon. Help the child to grasp the ribbon and pull it—for a spectacular demolition job. Be prepared to repeat the joke many times!

String-activated noisy mobiles

A Dancing Danglement

Quick

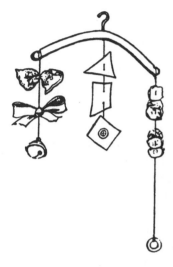

This is a mobile that does not rely on a draught to make it move. It is activated by 'baby power'. When the string is pulled, the mobile will bob about and set all the noisemakers jangling.

A coat-hanger is hung out of reach of the child, but where he can see it easily. An assortment of noisy objects and some colourful ones are tied to the hanger. These might include a bunch of bells, a string of foil milk bottle tops, a rattle, a tassel of brightly-coloured ribbons, cellophane sweet wrappers, tied in the middle to make them look like butterflies. Make about three strings of these with one considerably longer than the others. This is the one for the child to pull. Make it easy to hold by tying a ring or cotton reel to the end. Be sure the strings cannot slip off the hanger by either drilling holes for them or cutting notches in the top. On a plastic hanger, bind the strings in place with Sellotape.

A Bamboo Mobile

Long-lasting

This mobile can be used in two ways: in version 1, the mobile is hung out of reach (like the Dancing Danglement above), and the child pulls a string to make the sound; in version 2, as shown, it is hung within reach for a 'hands on' experience. In this case, the child can run his hands along the line of bamboo tubes to make them strike together. This mobile is weather-resistant, so is suitable for hanging outside on a veranda perhaps, or in the winter from the branches of a bare tree, where it could provide a welcome spot of colour in a dreary winter landscape.

Materials
- A length of broomstick or thick dowel for the hanging bar.
- Bamboo garden canes, say two.
- An old knitting needle.
- Paint. Acrylic is best, but poster will do.
- Polyurethane varnish.
- Thin nylon cord for suspending the support.

- Strong, thin thread for hanging the bamboo sections.
- Beads—optional, but they make the bamboo sections hang better and look pretty.
- Tools—a small saw, two drills, a craft knife, sandpaper.

Method

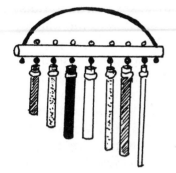

Divide the bamboo canes into separate sections by cutting about 10 mm above each joint. The sections will be different lengths and thicknesses. Discard any split or faulty ones and keep about eight to ten of the best. With a craft knife, scratch away all the waxy surface on the outside of each section. (Work away from yourself, and take care.) It is important to remove all the waxy surface or the paint will not stick properly, and will chip off when the sections knock together. Rub each section with sandpaper to ensure that the surface is smooth and clean. Drill a small hole, just large enough to take the hanging thread, down through the joint at the top of each section. Working from the open end of the cane, scratch out the pith in the middle with a knitting needle. Tap it on the table now and then and the loose pith will fall out. Hold the cane up to your eye, and you should now be able to see right through it. Poke the hanging thread through the hole in the top of the section and out through the bottom. Tie a very large knot on the end, or better still, thread it through a small bead to prevent it from pulling out through the hole in the joint. Paint all the bamboo sections in bright colours and, when they are dry, protect each with at least two coats of polyurethane varnish.

Now decide how you would like them to hang—perhaps graded by size, or alternately long and short?—and arrange them in a row. Leave a gap between each about the width of a cane, and measure the length of the row. Cut the broomstick (or dowel) hanger about 8 cm (3") longer than this measurement. Drill holes at appropriate intervals along it, one for each section of bamboo and one at each end for the suspending cord. Tie each bamboo section (with the cord already in it) to the hanger. If you use beads, thread one as a spacer between a section and the hanger, and perhaps one on the top (as in the illustration) to make sure the section will not drop off. Finally, attach the suspending cord and a pull string if you are making version 1.

A Ship's Bell Rattle

Quick

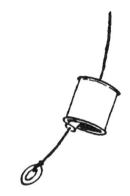

Any child who learns the knack of pulling the clapper of this strange bell sharply against its tin exterior will be instantly rewarded for his effort. The bell is made from an upturned treacle tin and the clapper is a large wooden bead, or a wooden brick with a hole drilled through it, or even a wooden cotton reel, if you happen to have such a rare treasure! First, thoroughly wash the treacle tin and dry it. Punch a small hole in the centre of the bottom. Push from the outside in, so that any jagged edges are inside the tin. Thread about 45 cm (18") of thick string or piping cord through the hole and decide on how much you need for the hanging loop and how much for the pull string. Then tie a large knot, which will disappear inside the tin (for it to rest on) and make another knot close to the bottom of the tin to prevent the cord from slipping inside. Thread the clapper onto the cord and tie a knot to prevent it from slipping off. Tie a ring to the end of the pull cord to make it easier to grasp. Decorate the outside of the tin with a strip of Fablon or paint it with Humbrol enamel. Tie the Ship's Bell within reach of the child and show him how to produce a surprising amount of decibels!

Note
This simple toy can also come in handy if a child is sick in bed. In these circumstances, a tiny hand bell, used to signal the need for attention, can easily be lost or dropped. Not so the Ship's Bell, which can be tied to the bed head.

Jumping Jacks

Long-lasting

Jumping Jacks are traditional toys, usually made in wood. They can only be activated if someone pulls the string.The one illustrated is made in cardboard. It combines movement with sound, and is jointed with paper fasteners—the kind with 'legs' that open out.

It is sensible to make a paper pattern first. This can help you to decide on the size and the shape of the pieces, and you can make sure your design will work well before you spend time on the cardboard version.

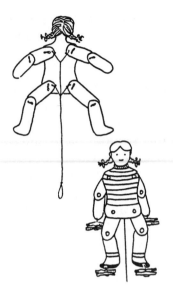

Before you begin, look at the illustration and work out the mechanics of making your Jack (or Jill) jump. Then draw the body with the head attached by a fairly thick neck (for strength). Cut out two sausage-shaped arms and decide on the best positions for them. They must swivel on the paper fasteners so as to be horizontal with the body when the connecting string is pulled fully down, and be almost hidden by the body when relaxed. Cut out the legs, also sausage-shaped, but larger than the arms and with suggested feet on the end.

When you are happy with your design, transfer the shapes to fairly thick cardboard and cut them out with a craft knife or Snips (really strong kitchen scissors similar to secateurs). Paint all the pieces. Fix on the limbs with paper fasteners, and string them as shown in the illustration. For an added attraction, tie a string of foil milk-bottle tops (with a button on the bottom of the string to stop them slipping off), to the hands and feet. Alternatively, tie on bells.

Hang your Jumping Jack against a plain wall if possible, and just out of a child's reach. The string must, of course, be within his grasp, so that he is in control and the Jumping Jack will dance to his bidding.

A Plywood Owl Jumping Jack

Long-lasting

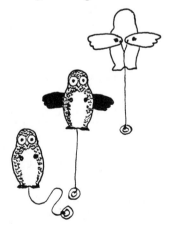

This toy works on the same principle as the one above, but only his wings move. For anyone with a fretsaw, it is easy to make, and the finished owl is very robust.

Make a paper pattern first. Draw the owl's head and body, making him about 30 cm (12") long. Give him large eyes and make him chubby, so that his wings will fold neatly behind his body when at rest. Draw his wings and try them out by fixing them in place with paper clips. Make sure they will flap nicely. Transfer the body and wing shapes to the plywood and cut them out. Sandpaper all the parts and paint in the eyes, beak and feathers. Drill two holes in each wing, one to fix it to the body and the other near the edge for the pull string. I joined my wings to the body with piping cord, knotting it in front of the body and behind the wings. Small nuts and bolts or rivets could be used. String up as shown in the illustration.

Note

After several weeks of heavy use, the piping cord on my owl stretched, and the wings started to rotate (!) causing a tangle at the back. Should this happen to you, the remedy is easy. Just glue a small strip of wood across the owl's shoulders to act as a stop.

A Tunnel Pop-up Toy

Quick

Marianne Willemsen-van Witsen

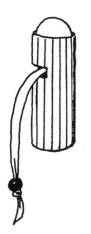

This toy can be fun for lots of children—the very active as well as the not so mobile. A ping-pong ball is hidden inside a tube. A sharp pull on the ribbon projects it out of the top, to be chased all over the room by the energetic. Pull the ribbon more gently to make the ball pop out less dramatically, and a skilful child, perhaps in a wheelchair, might be able to catch it before it reaches the floor.

Materials

- A ping-pong ball.
- A cardboard tube. Check that the tube is slightly wider than the ping-pong ball, for this has to move freely up and down inside it.
- Soft ribbon, about 2½ cm (1") wide and roughly four times the length of the tube.
- A bead for the end of the ribbon. This is optional, but makes it easier to grasp.
- PVA adhesive.
- Scissors (or a craft knife for adult use.)
- Decoration for the tube—paint, paper, Fablon or cloth.

Method

Cut a horizontal slit, like a letter box, in the cardboard tube, fairly near the top. Make it wide enough for the ribbon to slide through easily. Thread the ribbon through the slot to the inside of the tube. Pull it up and away from you, so that it comes out of the tube and over the edge. Stick it down the entire length of the 'back' of the tube. This will attach it firmly so that it will withstand plenty of pulling. Thread the free end of the ribbon through the bead and tie a knot.

Once the glue is dry, the toy is almost finished and ready for its trials. Try it out by pushing the ping-pong ball down inside the tube. It will sit in the sling of ribbon.

Pull the ribbon smartly, and the ball should shoot out of the top of the tube. If you have a problem, it could be because the tube has been slightly squashed, and the ball gets stuck. Reinforce the tube with strips of paper and glue, or find another one and start again! Perhaps the slot needs enlarging slightly, or even moving a little nearer the top of the tube.

When you are satisfied the toy is working well, decorate the tube.

A Pop-up Matchbox

Quick

Marianne Willemsen-van Witsen

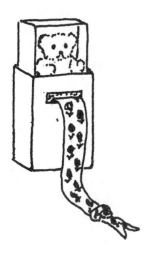

If you have already made the Tunnel Pop-up Toy, you will have no difficulty with this one. It works on the same principle. The action is slower and less dramatic, but this can be a definite advantage for those children who need a little time to focus their attention on something new. Pull the ribbon, and the tray of the matchbox will rise most of the way out of its cover to reveal its hidden treasure.

Materials
● A matchbox.
● A short length of ribbon, about 20 cm (8") wide
● A bead (optional).
● A decorative cover for the matchbox.
● Something to stick inside for the surprise—a tiny doll, a toy from a cracker or, perhaps, a familiar face cut from a photograph. If you have time and the inclination, you might create a little scene inside the tray, such as a window looking out onto a country scene, with dainty lace curtains and pot plants on the window sill.

Method
Remove the tray from the matchbox cover. Cut a slot about 2 cm (¾")from the top of the cover (wide enough to take the ribbon). If you make it nearer the top, the tray will come right out when the ribbon is pulled. If you make it further down, not enough of the tray will rise up. Even making a simple little toy like this can have its technical hazards!

Thread the ribbon through the slot to the inside of the cover, and pull it up and over the back. Stick it along the entire length of the back. Insert the tray gently so that it sits in the ribbon sling, then press it down. (The ribbon will shorten as the tray disappears inside the cover.) Tie a bead to the free end of the ribbon. Pull it gently to make sure the toy is working properly and the tray rises up as you expect. Take the tray out and decorate the part that will show. Then decorate the cover—the quickest way is to wrap it in coloured Sellotape, and this will also cover the abrasive strips at the side.

Pulling apart

Zanna's Plonk Pads

Quick

Zanna was a member of the Special Care Unit. She had a distressing habit of biting her thumb whenever she was left to her own devices. Her teacher tried various ways of keeping her hands occupied and away from her teeth, but success was patchy. The only sure solution was one-to-one attention, but with a room full of equally demanding children that was, of course, not easy. Zanna liked to pull at the Velcro fastening on the front of her jacket. This gave me a clue for a 'toy' which I hoped would keep her hands busy. I made a couple of small cushions like shoe-polishing pads, the right size to fit Zanna's hands. A long strip of Velcro was sewn down the centre of each pad. Now they could be endlessly pressed together, then pulled apart, making the rending sound Zanna liked so much. To make the pads easier to hold, a strip of elastic was sewn across the back of each. Zanna's fingers could be slipped under the elastic, which then rested across the backs of her hands. These 'Plonk Pads' met with success until the novelty wore off. They led to the invention of the next toy which has had an enthusiastic reception at the toy library!

Popper Balls

Long-lasting

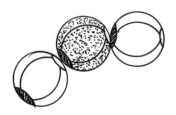

Imagine a bag full of small brightly-coloured felt balls, each with two Velcro spots attached . . . 'hooks' on the top, 'furry' on the bottom. Now the balls can be joined together in a long line, or formed into a circle to make a giant necklace (Perfectly safe to wear! If pulled it instantly falls apart!) The colours can be arranged in pairs, or as a sequence, and all the time the child can be joining them together and pulling them apart again. They can even be used as rewards for tasks completed.

The children of my experience like to see how long a line of Popper Balls they can collect before the working session is over.

Materials
- A small piece of cardboard for a template for a section of the ball.
- Felt in as many bright colours as possible.
- Velcoins. These are circles of Velcro, obtainable from any shop that sells aids for dressmakers. (Velcro spots will also do, but these are slightly smaller and do not stick together quite so easily.)
- Polyester filling.

Method
Each ball is made from six segments which are shaped like the petals of a flower (*see* p. 94). An easy way to make this shape is to draw a rectangle on your cardboard 3 cm (1¼") × 9 cm (3½"). Make a little mark at the mid-point of each side. Start at the mark in the middle of a short side. Draw a curved line to the opposite mark, touching the mark on the long side as you go. Draw the mirror image. Hopefully, the shape you have made resembles a petal! Use your template to mark out six segments for each ball. For the sake of appearances make sure your pencil lines will be on the inside of the ball. Pin the segments together. Hand sew all the seams, but leave a small opening in the last one. Stuff each ball just enough to make it a good shape, and close the gap. Avoid over-stuffing or the balls will be too heavy to stick together well. Sew a 'hooked' Velcoin to the North Pole and a 'furry' one to the South Pole. Make plenty of balls . . . and play can begin.

Unfortunately, these balls will not wash and may need a trip to the dry cleaners now and then. I think this disadvantage is outweighed by the ease of working in felt, and the gorgeous colours available. The balls need to be quite small, otherwise they are too heavy to stick together satisfactorily. I tried making them in cotton on the sewing machine, but found the short, curved seams very fiddly. Perhaps your sewing techniques are better than mine!

A Feely Caterpillar

Long-lasting

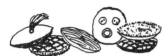

Here is another toy for pulling apart and putting together again. It consists of a series of small cushions which can be assembled to make a rather strange caterpillar. It has a face on the front and a *tail* on the back! (I know this makes it a creature unknown to man. The children won't object and as a toy it gives it a defined ending!) The segments can either be arranged in a sequence by texture or by colour. First comes the face. The back of that cushion matches (by texture or colour) the front of the next cushion . . . and so on all along the creature until the final cushion which will have the tail on the back of it.

Materials
Directions are given for the textured version.

- A saucer for a template.
- A collection of different materials to match by texture—say six, e.g. velvet, fur fabric, corduroy, etc.
- A pack of Velcoins.
- A small amount of polyester filling to stuff the cushions lightly.
- Scraps of felt or buttons for the features.
- A small amount of wool to make a tassel for the tail.

Method
Using the saucer as a template, draw two circles on the wrong side of each piece of fabric. Cut out the circles. Arrange them in pairs in a row in front of you. Take a circle from the first pair and give it a face. You could attach two buttons for eyes and a curtain ring for a mouth, or you could sew on felt features. Put the face back at the head of the row. Take its twin circle and sew a tassel to its centre. Wind the wool over all your fingers several times. Gently slip it off and bind the little hank you have made very firmly near one end. Cut the wool at the other end to make the tassel. Sew the loops at the bound end to the circle. Put this tail piece at the far end of the row. Take a circle from the next pair of textures and sew one half of a Velcoin to the centre. Pin it to the back of the face, wrong sides together for the moment

so that you can check how the sequence of textures works out. Sew the other half of the Velcoin to the matching circle. Back it with a circle from the next pair (Velcoin attached). Continue in this way, matching texture to texture, until you reach the tail. The sequence of textures should be AB-BC-CD-D . . . A. At this stage, it is sensible to check that the Velcro coupling also works and you have not inadvertently put two of the same kind on one segment of the caterpillar.

Now to make up the caterpillar. Start with the head. Remove the pins, put right sides together, tack, and sew most of the way round, leaving a gap for turning and stuffing. Turn, lightly stuff and close the gap. Continue like this all down the line of cushions. Join them together as you go to check that all is well.

A Spinner

Quick

Here is a toy for older children. There is a knack to making it work. It needs the use of both hands and average muscular strength. It is just a disc suspended in the centre of a loop of string. The disc can be set spinning by a pulling movement rather like using a chest expander! Children who can master the knack get hooked on it. It is made from a length of string, say 1 m (40") and a circle of thin ply, about 8–10 cm (3½—4") in diameter. Cut out the circle. Rule a line through the centre. On this line drill two holes, just large enough to take the string, and about 2 cm (¾") from the centre. Decorate both sides of the disc with a brightly-coloured pattern. Thread the string through both holes and tie the ends together to make a loop. Hold the loop with both hands and make sure the disc is in the centre. Twirl it round to twist up the string. Then move your hands sharply apart to stretch out the string and set the disc spinning. At the critical moment, relax your hands so that the spinning continues and the string twists round the opposite way. Stretch out again, then relax . . . and so on, to keep the disc spinning. This can take some practice.

Grasp and release

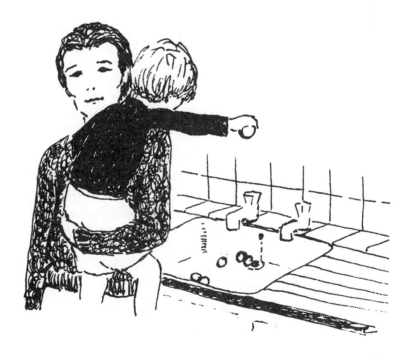

The simple act of gripping and then letting go—so easy and automatic for us—can be a hard movement for some children to master. As with all skills, the more play activities that can be devised to back up the therapy sessions, the more quickly the child is likely to acquire this essential movement. The child in the illustration must be having fun dropping the ping-pong ball into a sink full of water. Hopefully, a brother or sister is standing by to retrieve the ball and help him to repeat the action over and over again for as long as his interest lasts. This simple game can easily lead on to the one below, then to other 'grasp and release' activities, such as playing with posting boxes and the ideas for 'stacking' and 'throwing and catching' which follow.

Drop It In

Instant

Pam Courtney,
Teacher

Pam has a collection of containers which she stores in a large cardboard box. These include a cake tin, plastic bowls of different sizes, a coffee tin, a wooden box, a plastic ice cream tub, etc. She also has a variety of objects, which can be put into them: plastic and metal spoons, pasta shells, cotton reels, fir cones, stones, woolly balls—anything that can ultimately be sorted into groups. At first, the children just put anything into anything! Dropping a metal spoon into a cake tin will make a lovely clatter, and besides being fun, of course practises the action of grasping and releasing. The next stage is to put all the cotton reels in one container, the pasta shells in another, and so on.

A Simple Posting Box with Only One Hole

Instant

This toy can be a winner for any child who is just starting to take an interest in putting one thing inside another. This can happen at any age from about ten months upwards. As well as being good fun, cheap, and easy to make, it can be used as an introduction to more complicated commercial posting boxes.

All you need is a tin with a plastic lid, such as a coffee tin, and a supply of cotton reels to post inside. The tin should be as large as possible. Make sure the lip is 'rolled' (not sharp) and that the cotton reels are all the same size. Use one as a template to mark a circle in the centre of the lid. Cut this out—with scissors or with a heated needle embedded in a cork, so that you can hold it comfortably. The hole should be slightly larger than the reel so that it will drop through easily. Check there are no jagged edges to the circle. (A rub with sandpaper will remove them.)

To make this simple toy more attractive, paint the tin and reels with Humbrol enamel. One coat should be sufficient, and you will end up with a colourful toy with twice the child appeal.

At the Sense Centre (for deaf/blind children), the teachers use a series of simple one-hole posting boxes. They consider the special needs of the children with flaccid hands. The size of the hole in the lid is carefully controlled, so that pushing an object through it requires some effort. The children begin with a ping-pong ball. When they are successful, the ping-pong ball falls into the tin with a satisfying clonk. As they become adept at this, they move on to another tin with a smaller hole which will just accept a wooden bead. Next comes a third for posting plastic hair curlers. These present a new problem. They need to be up-ended before they will fit into the hole. The sound and feel of the little plastic bristles on the sides of the curlers rubbing against the edge of the hole can set the teeth of an adult on edge but, of course, the children love it!

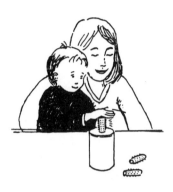

Posting Acorns in a Bottle

Instant

Susan Myatt, Parent, Kingston-upon-Thames Toy Library

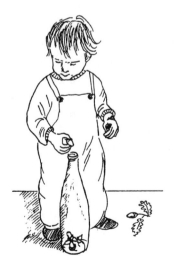

All children like to play with natural objects and things from the adult world. These are the nuts and bolts of our environment, and through them children learn about the world in which they live. Picture in your mind's eye a two-year-old totally absorbed in fitting the lids on heavy saucepans. A year later, he may be splashing in the puddles or scuffing up the Autumn leaves, while at home his big sister is playing at weddings, draping herself in an old net curtain and wearing her mother's shoes. Some children cannot share in these delights, but *if* you are reading this in the Autumn, and *if* you live near an oak tree, and *if* your child has reached the 'posting' stage, here is a chance to bring the outside world nearer to him, and let him practise his new-found skill into the bargain—and all completely free!

All you need is a bag full of acorns (perhaps you can collect them together) and a plastic bottle. If you want your child to practise fine finger movements, choose a bottle with a neck just wide enough to accept an acorn end on. Now sit back and watch his delight as he sees the bottle gradually filling up because of his own skilful efforts.

Posting Drinking Straws in a Bottle

Instant

Lorraine Crawford's little daughter

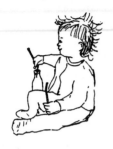

This idea is similar to the one above, but it has two advantages. It can be set up in seconds, so really is *instant*, and it does not rely on a seasonal crop of acorns. Lorraine's small daughter was playing on the kitchen floor when an empty milk bottle caught her attention. Here was an unusual container just waiting to be filled! She tried to push a spoon down the neck, but in spite of all her efforts, the bowl remained outside. She searched around for something else to try. She had instant success with a pot of pencils, but even better was a bunch of drinking straws someone thoughtfully provided. These were long and bendy, and needed to be lined up with the neck of the bottle before they could be dropped inside.

A Custom-Made Posting Box

Quick

Peter was a lad with cerebral palsy. Like many other such children, he had great difficulty in letting go of an object once his fingers were clasped tightly round it. His Physiotherapist asked me to devise a toy which could encourage him to pick something up, extend his arm, and then release the object. What seemed to be needed was an oversize posting box with only one hole. After a quick survey of all the scrap materials available, a plastic sweet jar was chosen to be the container. This had a wide neck, which made a good target to aim for. The jar was also transparent, so seeing the results of his efforts as he gradually filled it up should give Peter some 'job satisfaction'.

The first problem was how to keep the jar stable, for it was large, and in its empty state very light and easily knocked over. The solution was simple. A few stones were placed in the bottom of the jar and were covered with Polyfilla, mixed to a consistency just sloppy enough to settle between them. When this had set, the jar had a permanently weighted base. Now all that was needed was something suitable to drop into it. Tennis balls were the ideal size to fit Peter's hand but, when using these, his jerky movements would scatter them to the four corners of the room. The answer proved to be a generous supply of our old friends, soft woolly balls, which we stored in a plastic bowl resting on a Dycem mat.

For anyone who missed out on making soft woolly balls in their youth, this is how it is done. Cut two identical circles from card—the Cornflakes packet will do. Make the diameter about 10 cm, (4"). Cut a hole in the centre of each, about 4 cm (1½") wide. Put the circles together and wind wool over the edge and up through the middle, gradually working your way all round the ring. At this stage, the ball resembles a ring doughnut. As the hole gradually fills up, you will need a needle threaded with wool to finish the winding. If you hold the ring up to your eye and you cannot see through it, this part of the job is finished.

Now take a pair of sharp-pointed scissors and, at one point on the circumference of the circle, snip the wool until you come to the cardboard. Poke the scissors between the two card circles, and continue cutting all round. You now have lots of strands of wool sticking out each side of the cardboard circles. Pull the cardboard circles a little way apart. Using strong button thread, bind *tightly* round the wool *between* the cardboard circles, finishing off with a sturdy knot. Snip the cardboard circles and pull them away. Fluff up the wool to make the ball a good shape, and trim off any odd ends.

Posting Pictures in a Shoe Box

Quick

Ann Macpherson,
Portage Worker

Look at the picture of the cross-section of this easily-made (and cheap) posting box. You will see that it differs from the usual commercial ones where shapes are posted through the appropriate holes, only to be seen again when the boxes are opened. In this case, the letters posted inside disappear, travel down the cardboard slide, then pop out of the slot at the bottom of the

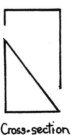
Cross-section

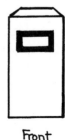
Front

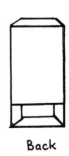
Back

back! This feature makes it attractive to the average toddler and most are happy to repeat the action over and over again. For her 'letters' Ann uses pictures from Ladybird Books, mounted on card and protected with clear sticky-backed plastic. The pictures are selected for their speech value, and their appeal for the special child with whom she is working. She deliberately cuts the posting slot so that the cards will only be accepted end on. Now the child must work out how to send each one on its way. For a child with a visual impairment, Ann might highlight the slot by edging it with strips of difraction paper (p. 7). Otherwise, it is made prominent with a simple black (felt pen) edging. Before each picture is about to be posted, it can be named and discussed. As well as helping to improve a child's hand function, this toy can also be used to enlarge and consolidate his vocabulary. Sometimes the box is placed between two children, one to post and one to retrieve.

As a home visitor, Ann appreciates a toy which is fairly small and easy to transport. In its raw state a shoebox is likely to have a limited life, but strengthen it by fixing on the lid with sticky tape and covering it all (except the slot!) with layers of paper and paste and it will withstand many more play sessions. Make it look more like a real post box by applying a coat of red paint and, maybe, a final protective covering of polyurethane varnish.

Plink Plonk

Instant

This simple idea could persuade a child to use both hands, grasp and release, (post) look, (aim) and listen! How's that for incidental therapy? It will probably not hold a child's interest for very long, but as the game is simplicity itself to set up, it is worth a try!

All you need is a fairly wide and long cardboard tube, a collection of items to post down it, and a tin to catch them all at the bottom. Should you not have a cardboard tube to hand, just roll up a newspaper (or two), starting from the folded edge and fix the loose edges together with Sellotape. You should now have a fairly sturdy tube. Find a biscuit (or baking) tin and assemble the collection of postable items. Be imaginative here, and take the chance to introduce shapes, textures and common objects of different weights. All should land in the tin with a satisfying thud! Perhaps this short list will start you thinking. Toys, and bits of toys, e.g. bricks, stacking rings, fir-cones, cotton reels, beanbags, rolled up socks, plastic egg cups, spoons (various), stones (rough or smooth as appropriate).

Drainpipe Skittles

Instant

Brian Spencer,
Remedial Gymnast,
The Manor Hospital

Brian worked with teenagers who were in wheelchairs. Some had difficulty in using their hands efficiently. The game of skittles was a firm favourite with them all, and was made playable for those unable to bowl in the normal way by providing them with a length of drainpipe. Using this simple aiming device, all the player had to do was to release the ball when he judged the drainpipe to be pointing in the right direction. It would travel down the pipe and, hopefully, scatter the skittles. Brian found that a sweet placed on top of a particular skittle considerably increased the player's concentration—and his enjoyment, for if he knocked it off he was entitled to eat it!

Feeding a Face

Quick

This activity is very popular with the under-fives at our local Assessment Centre. As you can imagine from its title, it involves posting 'food' through the open mouth of a cheerful face painted on the side of a cardboard carton. Of course, it encourages the posting action, but it also leads to plenty of conversation about the food on offer. The children often learn new words and consolidate them when that particular food is on the menu again. Children, who find it very difficult to grasp, feed the face with real food, such as an apple or carrot, or 'pretend' food made from papier mâché (buns, biscuits, fish fingers, sausages, chips, etc.) Other children feed the face with *pictures* of food mounted on fairly thick card. A quick flip through a glossy magazine will usually produce some delectable menus. As well as choosing their favourite food, some children enjoy the joke of making up revolting mixtures, like cabbage and strawberries or eggs and jam!

Note

This activity makes a good preparation for the next stage—to post letters and cards in a bright red model post box. For the younger children their 'mail' will be pictorial or just scribble, but older children like to send each other, or members of staff, little notes and, of course, homemade cards for birthdays and Christmas.

Stacking

Children with poor hand control seldom play with a stacking toy from choice. It can be so difficult and frustrating for them to try to pile one object on top of another, and to place something over a rod may be even more difficult. However, the usual stacking toys on the shop shelves are not the only way of practising this useful skill. Here are some alternatives.

Stack Anything

Instant

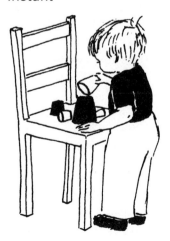

- Saucepans
- Flower pots
- Egg cups
- Cotton reels
- Limpet shells (difficult)
- Stones with a flat surface, washed smooth by the sea—painted as an optional extra
- Yogurt pots or polystyrene cups
- Christmas cards. Place the first one opened out as though standing on the mantlepiece. Lie the second one horizontally across it, stand the third one on top of that ... and so on, until the whole lot topple down!

Ideas contributed by Pam Courtney, Christine Cousins and Kanji Watenabi.

Stacking Socks

Quick

This simple stacking toy is a great confidence builder, and also requires the child to grasp and let go. Most households acquire a little collection of toddler's socks, which have lost their partners. When you have lost all hope of a happy reunion, they can be given a new life as a splendid stacking toy. Lightly fill each one so that it is easy for the child to grasp. Avoid over-stuffing or the socks will not flop nicely on top of each other. The choice of stuffing is up to you. You can even adjust the weight of each sock, if that would be helpful to the child in question. I use polyester stuffing for lightness, dried peas or rice (won't wash!) for a medium weight and fish grit for a heavier filling. Stitch firmly across the top of each sock to keep the contents safely inside, and the child can pile them, however inaccurately, one on top of the other until the supply runs out.

Higher and Higher

Quick

Lekotek Korea,
The Toy Library,
Seoul

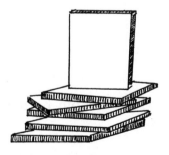

Here is a more conventional stacking toy. It is nothing more than a collection of flat wooden slabs, but it really works! The slabs are made from thick ply or MDF (medium density fibreboard) with all the edges nicely sanded to give a smooth, splinter-free surface. The rectangular slabs are piled up in the usual way but, because of their shape, they do not need to be placed precisely on top of each other. A child, who cannot manage to stack cube-shaped bricks, will have a good chance of success with these. Without being too accurate, it is possible to make a really high tower, which should give the child a pleasant glow of achievement. On the way, he will have practised his hand-eye coordination and the skill of grasping and releasing.

Alternative Version, Not Using Wood

Quick

If the idea of 'Higher and Higher' appeals to you, but you do not have the facilities for making it as suggested by the toy library in Korea, try making a less durable version with small, flat boxes such as kitchen match boxes (the large size), or any other suitable packaging. Strengthen each box with a filling of small, crunched-up pieces of newspaper. Make sure it stays a good shape.

Bind it with sticky tape—Sellotape, parcel tape, masking tape, etc. You can either leave it at that, or spend a little more time decorating each box with paint or gift wrapping paper.

Small, Very Light Bricks

Long-lasting

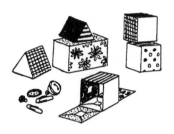

Easy to make, but time consuming! These bricks are particularly suitable for 'frail' children, and for any child with flaccid hands and a poor grip. A set was made for Rupert, a little boy of one-and-a-half, who had a rare skin condition which affected his hands. Because of the tender nature of his skin, it was essential for him to have light-weight playthings which would cause the least friction. Spotlessly clean toys were also a necessity. These bricks can go in the washing machine and wash beautifully at a low temperature. They are made from squares of plastic cut from a margarine or ice cream tub. Each square is covered with fabric, patchwork fashion, and six are stitched together to form a cube. Rupert was interested in anything that made a noise, so his bricks had either a few foil milk bottle tops, small buttons, paper clips or bells inside them. He used them for stacking and building, and as a sound discrimination game, grouping together all those with the same contents.

Materials
- Plenty of plastic tubs and boxes. If the plastic is thin and bendy, use it double. There will be a lot of wastage, because only the flat areas are useful.
- Scraps of material. Cotton is best.
- Stiff card or ply for a template; size at your discretion—5 cm square (2") is suggested. This is too large to be swallowed, but it is a convenient size for small hands.
- Noisemakers if you want your bricks to rattle. Avoid rice, lentils, etc., as these will not wash!

Method
To make one brick . . .
Use the template and cut six squares from the flat parts of the plastic containers. Lay one square onto the material. Cut round it, allowing at least 1 cm seam allowance all round. Fold the top and bottom allowance

over the plastic and lace the edges together with a long zigzag tacking stitch. Turn in the other two sides and also zigzag them together, making the corners as neat as possible. Repeat for the other five squares.

Hold two squares together, with right sides face to face, and oversew along one edge. Make a few extra stitches at the corners for added strength. Open them out and add two more squares, making a strip of four. Add the two remaining squares, one each side of the strip to make a cross. Fold it up to make a cube. Join together all the unstitched sides by oversewing them, or using ladder stitch. If your brick is intended to rattle, remember to insert the noisemaker before you close the last seam. Make as many more bricks as you need.

Note
It is possible to make these bricks in a variety of shapes, e.g. cut two squares, 5 × 5 cm (2 × 2") and four rectangles 5 × 10 cm, (2 × 4") and you have a double-sized brick. For a ridged roof, cut three squares (or rectangles) and two equilateral triangles, base 5 cm. For a pyramid, cut one square and four triangles.

Foam Stacking Bricks

Quick

These are about the size of a house brick, or a little larger. Inside the brightly-coloured fabric covers are blocks of plastic foam used in upholstery. The plastic foam keeps its shape well. It is also fairly soft, so that a child who finds it hard to pick up a brick in the usual way can handle this set by using a pinching movement and squeezing into the plastic foam. Because of their light weight, they can be handled by children with less than normal strength. Their large size, and the way they can be used to make spectacular structures, seems to make them attractive to all children who are at the 'stacking stage'.

The plastic foam can be bought, in various thicknesses and density, at specialist shops dealing in upholstery materials and at street markets. It is sold by length and is easy to cut into any size you want. An electric carving knife is the best tool for the job but, failing that, a serrated bread knife will do. Each block of plastic foam is then fitted into an attractive cotton cover. This should be a tight fit so that the finished brick remains a good shape. I find it saves time in the end to make templates the exact sizes for the ends, top (and bottom) and sides of the brick. (Size at your discretion.) Then all you have to do is to place the templates on the fabric, leaving a space between them for the seam allowance. Draw round each template in pencil. The pencil lines show where to stitch the seams, so remember to cut outside them. Repeat the process to make as many shapes as you require to cover the number of bricks you have in mind. Cut out all the shapes (two ends and four sides for each brick) and with right sides together pin along the appropriate pencil lines. Stitch along the seams, leaving one open (so that you can insert the foam). Turn your cover right side out and stuff in the foam block making sure it goes into all the corners to make a good shape. A knitting needle is useful for this job. Close the open seam by hand.

Adapting Wooden Bricks

Quick

Audrey Stevenson,
Toy Designer

Audrey had a friend who taught young children with Cerebral Palsy. She wanted them to learn to stack one brick on top of another but, because of their jerky movements, they found this task very difficult. The foam bricks described above would not be suitable for some of the children in the group. They were inclined to dribble, so their toys needed frequent washing. Audrey came up with the bright idea of sticking Velcro to all the surfaces of wooden bricks so that, once they were placed even approximately in position, they would stick together. She made two sets of bricks, using black and white squares of Velcro. One set had black 'hooks' and white 'furry' squares and the textures were reversed on the other set, so no Velcro was wasted! This idea worked well because the children soon realised they must always put white on black. If the Velcro had not been in highly contrasting colours, the children would have found it difficult to sort out the 'furry' surfaces from the 'hooked' ones. (I was tempted to use this principle with another group of older children until I remembered I had spent some considerable time encouraging them to match like colours in many different ways. I feared that suddenly asking them to match black to white might muddle them up!)

A Tropical Aquarium

Long-lasting

Mr Poediangga

As a student, Mr Poediangga attended a course at HEARU (Handicap, Education and Aids Research Unit) and invented this clever stacking toy.

Three chunky fish locate over short lengths of dowel fitted into a base board. (For even more stability, this can be clamped to the table.) The thickness of the wood makes the pieces easy to handle and, of course, each fish is attractively painted in brilliant colours.

Materials
- A base board, say 350 cm × 150 cm × 20 mm (14 × 6 × ¾").
- Three short lengths of dowel, rounded at the top.
- Wood glue.
- A piece of 38 mm (10") soft wood for the fish.
- Paint.
- Polyurethane varnish for protection.

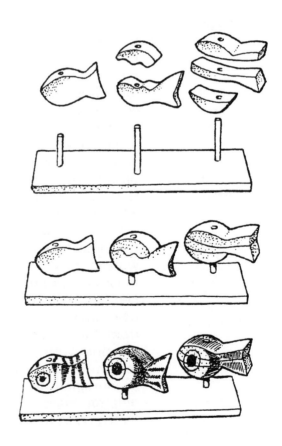

Method

Look at the illustration and drill holes in the base board for the dowel rods. Glue them in place. Cut out the outlines of the fish. Drill a hole through each, slightly larger than the diameter of the dowel for an easy fit. Leave one fish intact, divide the second into two pieces and the last one into three. Sandpaper all the pieces. Paint them as gaudily as possible, then cover with at least two coats of polyurethane varnish.

Build a Town

Quick

Now for the ultimate in building activities! Do you ever organise a festivity for older children where you are fortunate enough to have that rare luxury, plenty of space? If so, the following tale may interest you.

Every year the school for children with learning difficulties where I was then working held a Fun Day. Children, parents and staff all trooped out to the playing field, watched (or took part in) the fancy dress parade, shared a mammoth picnic, then dispersed to the edges of the field to take part in all the activities on offer. Some headed for the candy floss, others fished for plastic ducks in a paddling pool or tried their luck at the hoop-la or lucky dip . . . or whatever else took their fancy.

My contribution to the jollification was to supply a huge quantity of cardboard boxes which had been

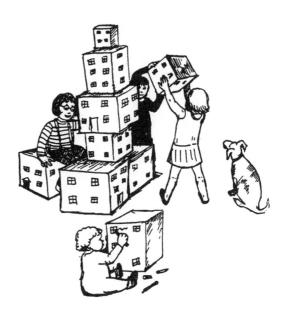

transformed into giant building bricks. For weeks the senior pupils had been sticking down the flaps and covering the boxes with left-over dregs of emulsion paint donated by staff and parents. The result of all this industry was an enormous heap of multicoloured cubes just waiting for someone to build them into something!

As it happened, the first visitor to my patch was a very tall lad. He spent a happy five minutes building a high tower of single boxes. Luckily he realised the biggest should go at the bottom, so he managed to achieve a monumental edifice, even taller than himself. It was visible for some distance and soon attracted other would-be builders. Throughout the afternoon, walls, tower blocks, enclosures and 'ruins' were made. All this involved a great deal of thought, bending and stretching, balancing, etc., but above all, judging by the reactions of both builders and spectators, it helped to put the fun in 'Fun Day'!

Throwing and catching

Simple ball games are often a child's first experience of playing an organised game with someone else. In the initial stages a grown-up needs to be involved. While the play lasts, child and adult have each other's undivided attention, and both can find this very enjoyable.

AIMING GAMES

All ball and beanbag games are excellent for encouraging children to look, hold and let go. It is not hard to invent a simple 'to' and 'fro' game to meet the requirements of almost any child. When a baby can sit unsupported, he may be ready for the simplest of all ball play. Just aim for his hand and slowly roll a large and colourful ball across the floor towards it. When he 'catches' the ball, he will probably want to put it in his mouth and generally explore it. After a while, he will be willing to give it up for the joy of having it bowled to him again. Sitting him with his legs apart, forming a sort of harbour, will make it easier to field the ball. The next stage is for the child to return the ball to you. Already he is starting to learn a basic ball skill as he tries to aim in a certain direction. When he realises how difficult this is, I guess his sense of humour will come to the fore, and he will have more fun deliberately mis-aiming and making you chase after the ball!

Beanbags

At the early stages of teaching a child to throw and catch, there is a lot to be said for using beanbags instead of balls. They are easier to grasp, nestle into the hand nicely and do not roll away or bounce. They usually measure about 10 × 15 cm (4 × 6") but the proportions can easily be scaled up or down for large or small hands. As well as rectangular, they can also be made square, circular or triangular. My favourite shape is like a starfish. This not only looks attractive but, on the practical side, the five points of the star drape nicely over the child's hand as he catches it.

A beanbag can be made in any material strong enough to withstand hard wear. Rip-stop nylon is perhaps the best of all. This is used in making kites, etc., is seemingly indestructible and comes in brilliant colours. For the cost of the postage, a kite-making factory once sent me a parcel of offcuts, and I have also found this fabric at my local Scrap Bank.

The filling, which comes about halfway up the bag, usually consists of dried peas or rice. Both make for a good, floppy beanbag, but will not wash. Where washability is an issue, use fish grit from the pet shop. This filling is heavier than those above, which can be an advantage for some children with 'butter fingers'.

Special Beanbags

Quick

Monica Taylor,
Toy Librarian,
The Rix Toy Library

Monica designed some unusual beanbags for a particular group of lively teenagers. They all found throwing and catching difficult, so any game played with a round, fast-moving and elusive ball, was not enjoyable for them. Monica made large, cuddly cylindrical beanbags, about 30 cm (12") long. These were filled with polystyrene packaging chips, which gave a pleasant rustly sound when squeezed. They were also very light, and therefore harmless if badly aimed! The teenagers were not interested in tearing the bags so, played with under supervision, they were quite safe for use with this group. Polystyrene chips are dangerous if eaten, and should never be put into bags made for young children or older, stronger ones who may rip the covers.

Balls

A visit to a toy shop will provide you with plenty of choice, but you may be looking for a ball which has sober habits and will not roll too fast. In this case the best idea is often an evening of DIY! Here are some suggestions for slow-moving balls:

A Woolly Ball

Easy, but time consuming

Turn to p. 79 and find the instructions for making the woolly balls to post in the 'Custom-made Posting Box'. For ball play, make your woolly ball quite large—suggested minimum diameter of the card circles about 20 cm (9"). The holes in the centres will then be about 8 cm (3") diameter. Use double knitting wool, wind evenly over the two thicknesses of card, and you will soon fill up the hole. As with the smaller balls, a needle threaded with wool will be necessary to complete the job and close the hole. Finish off the ball as before.

Note
Making a ball like this can be an excellent way of using up any odd lengths of wool. Go for bright colours and include some dark ones to give contrast. Avoid too many pastel shades as this ball will spend most of its life on the floor. Providing it is tightly tied together in the centre, it will wash well, but takes a long time to dry.

A Felt or Fabric Ball

Long-lasting

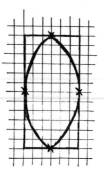

The way to make a ball in segments, like the 'Popper Balls' in the section on 'Pulling Apart' has already been described on p. 72. Scale up the template to the size you want. Omit the Velcoins applied to their North and South poles. Replace them with circles of felt—to neaten the top and bottom of the ball. Stuff it fairly lightly and it will not roll too quickly.

Note

If you want your ball to withstand a busy life, use a strong fabric for the cover. If it is likely to be soon outgrown, go for the easier option and use felt. This will not fray, so the seams will not need oversewing, but it can split, wear thin, or even have holes picked in it by busy little fingers and, worst of all, it does not wash well. All these disadvantages may be outweighed by its bright colours and its easiness to sew.

A Patchwork Ball

Long-lasting

Betty Lewis,
Toymaker for the
Kingston-upon-Thames
Toy Library

Betty makes attractive soft balls with bells inside, which go down well with the toy library babies and toddlers. They are time-consuming to make, but the end results are very attractive and excellent 'first balls'. I am assuming that this ball will be made by those who already enjoy patchwork and are familiar with the technique. The ball is made from twelve five-sided patches. As these are oversewn together, edge to edge, mosaic fashion, they become the curved surface of the ball. (Think of the multiple mirror facets of a disco ball reduced to a mere twelve shapes, and you have a rough idea of the finished toy.)

Materials

- Cardboard to make a template for the patches. Either trace off the one illustrated (diagram a), which will give you a ball of about 7 cm (3") diameter or, if you want a larger one and are good at geometry, scale it up (see diagram b).
- Stiff paper for the patches.
- Small pieces of cotton—or similar fabric. Accentuate the mosaic nature of the ball by using different colours or patterns.

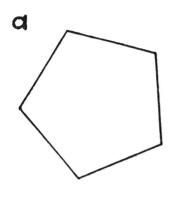

- Embroidery thread to herringbone stitch over the seams between the patches when the ball is completed (optional).
- A cat ball with a bell inside—from the pet shop.
- Polyester fibre for the stuffing

Method

Using the cardboard template, cut out (accurately!) twelve paper shapes. Before covering them with fabric, you may like to work out a colour scheme, or you could go for the easy option and make every shape different! As an experienced patchworker, you will have your own ideas about this! Choose one shape to be the centre of the top of the ball. Working on the wrong side, join five shapes to it to make a dome, like a skull cap with a zigzag edge. Make a similar dome for the bottom of the ball. Still working on the wrong side, oversew them together, most of the way round. Leave a gap for turning the ball the right side out and for inserting the cat ball and the stuffing. Close the gap. If you are fond of sewing, add a finishing touch by covering all the seams with herringbone or feather stitch worked in embroidery thread.

Some games using beanbags and balls

Aunt Sally

Quick

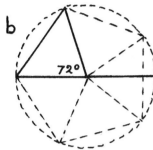

This throwing game is suitable for a group of children of mixed ages and ability. A sizeable cardboard box from the supermarket has a cheerful face painted on one side. The mouth is cut away to make a large hole through which beanbags can be thrown. A bell is suspended from the roof of the box, like a giant epiglottis. Every time a beanbag sails through the mouth, the bell rings to signal success! If necessary, a handicapping system can be agreed upon, with the more able children standing further from the target.

Toss in the Bin

Instant

This game is even easier to organise. Put a grocery carton or waste paper basket on the floor. Let the child stand fairly close at first, and throw in the beanbags. As skill increases, he stands further away. This game also comes in handy at clearing up time—put the beanbags away and play it with all the spilt Lego bricks!

Throw and Catch

Instant

Christine Cousins,
Educational
Psychologist

This game is the reverse of the one above. In this case, you do the throwing, while the child receives your missiles in a cardboard carton. This needs to be held firmly in both hands. Throw in objects of different weights. These should land on the bottom with a rewarding thud.

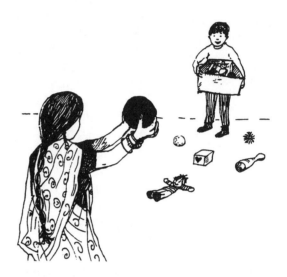

Another Target Game for Energetic Children

Instant

Roy McConkey,
Vice-President,
National Association
of Toy and Leisure
Libraries

In one of his lectures, Dr McConkey, a worldwide authority on play for people with special needs, suggested an instant throwing game which is packed full of activity. It can be played by two people, at any time, anywhere, for all it requires is a carrier bag and a modest supply of scrap paper. The paper is folded into paper darts, and one player aims these at a carrier bag held open by the other. The bag man aims to catch as many darts as possible. Remembering the erratic flight of most paper darts, the catcher must anticipate the course of the approaching missile and move nimbly to trap it in his bag.

Squeezing

Here is another hand movement encouraged by therapists as a way of strengthening a child's grip. Everyday living can provide plenty of practice through simple actions. Here are a few examples.

- Sqeezing the water out of the bath sponge.
- 'Shooting' the soap—squeezing it so that it shoots through the bath water (expensive on the soap, but a certain way to ensure clean hands!)
- Playing with a squeaky toy.
- Playing with playdough (recipes on pp. 99/100).

If you are looking for something a little more sophisticated try these ideas.

Squeezing Icing through an Icing Bag

Almost Instant

This activity is best indulged in just before bath time! If *you* like icing your child's birthday cake, why not mix up some softer icing and let *her* have a go? Provide some plain biscuits or even some strips of bread or toast, and her artistic efforts can be eaten later when the icing is firm. A word of warning. If the top of the icing bag is not firmly closed, you will soon discover that the mixture inside will backfire. Do not fill the bag too full. Roll the top over several times (like the paper bag in the vacuum cleaner) and secure it with bulldog clips (p. 11).

An Aromatic Puff Bottle

Very Quick

This is made from a plastic washing-up liquid bottle. Cut off the stopper. Remove the nozzle and wash the bottle out thoroughly. Shake the water out of it as best you can. Put in a tissue or some cotton wool balls sprinkled with a few drops of perfume or food flavouring. Replace the nozzle. The child can now practise her squeezing action by puffing a delectable smell in her own face or that of any responsive adult. The Puff Bottle will look more like a real toy if it is decorated with Humbrol enamel, which sticks well to the plastic and will not crack with squeezing. Alternatively, wrap it in a strip of material such as fur fabric or corduroy. Before applying the fabric, roughen the outside of the bottle with sandpaper to help the adhesive to stick—PVA is suitable—but some stitches over the join are necessary to keep this cover firmly in place and to prevent the child from picking it off. If you wish to change the smell in the bottle, it must first be given another good wash. An alternative smell might be a strong-smelling herb or spice, wrapped in a little bundle and forced through the neck of the bottle before the nozzle is replaced.

Divers in a Bottle

Quick

Daniel Hart,
Student on Work
Experience in a
Special School

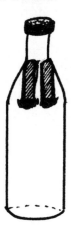

I met Daniel when he was working with a group of teenagers with severe learning difficulties. It was a wet day. At playtime the children were confined to the classroom. Daniel produced his water-filled bottle complete with two divers. As he squeezed the sides of the transparent plastic bottle, the divers sank gracefully to the bottom. When he stopped squeezing, they bobbed up to the top again. He soon attracted a small group of children all eager to try it. For one girl the fascination of this toy lasted the whole of playtime. She watched her friends play with it, and when their interest waned, she seized the bottle. She soon discovered how to make the divers plummet to the bottom. Then she began to experiment. She placed her hands on different parts of the bottle and squeezed with more or less pressure to see how the divers would react. (An early success for Daniel.)

Materials
- Transparent plastic bottle with cap, e.g. a fruit squash bottle.

- Two empty fountain pen ink cartridges for the divers.
- A small lump of Plasticine or Blu-tac.
- Water.

Method
Cut off the pricked ends of the cartridges. Wash them out. Seal the open ends with a blob of Plasticine. Fill the bottle with water. Insert the divers. Replace the cap on the bottle.

Note
When I copied this excellent squeezing toy, I found the amount of Plasticine used was critical. Be too generous and your divers will plunge straight to the bottom and stay there. Nothing for it but to empty out all the water and start again! If you do not use enough Plasticine, no amount of squeezing will induce your divers to perform. To allow a little time for scientific experimentation, this toy is classified *Quick* rather than *Instant*!

RECIPES FOR PLAYDOUGH

There are several ways of making playdough. Which one you choose may depend on the contents of your store cupboard! If mixed properly, all will make a pliable mixture. Those with a little oil in the recipe make the smoothest dough. Wrapped in a plastic bag, or stored in a screwtopped jar, they will keep in the fridge for about a week. On damp days the salt in the playdough may tend to make it sticky. Just add a little more flour. If your playdough cracks and does not hold together, it is too dry. Add a few more drops of water and mix them in well. Do not use playdough with a child who has cuts or broken skin on his hands. The salt in the dough will sting.

Recipe One
(The easiest)

- 1 large cup plain flour
- ½ cup salt
- A little water

Add the water very gradually and mix everything together until you get a pastry-like consistency.

Recipe Two

- 2 cups plain flour
- 1 cup salt
- 1 cup water (with food colouring or powder paint perhaps)
- 2 tablespoons cooking oil

Put all the ingredients in a bowl and mix together thoroughly.

Recipe Three

- 3 teacups plain flour
- 1½ cups cooking salt
- 3 teacups water
- 6 teaspoons cream of tartar
- 1 teaspoon cooking oil

Put everything in a saucepan and mix it all together. Stir it over a low heat until it all binds together and comes away from the sides of the pan. Leave it to cool.

Recipe Four

- ½ cup cornflour
- 1 cup salt
- ½ cup water

Blend everything together in a saucepan Cook over a low heat until the mixture thickens, stirring all the time to avoid lumps. Leave to cool.

Pinching

The title of this section might well be thought of as an anti-social activity and one definitely not to be encouraged between small children! In fact, 'pinching'—making the thumb and a finger work in opposition to each other—is a very useful action and, without it, the ability to perform many daily activities becomes very difficult—or even impossible. For example, it is essential for picking up small objects, for doing up a button, and with two fingers in opposition to the thumb, for holding a pencil. Try putting the key in the lock without using your thumb—and the point will be made!

If a child finds it difficult to make his fingers and thumb work in this way, the choice of suitable and interesting toys will help. As always, the golden rule is to 'begin where the child is at'. Start with toys that can be grasped—if only by the whole hand—and then gradually lessen the size of the toy as finger and thumb are able to work more closely together.This was our approach to Jamie, a three-year-old toy library member with learning difficulties and floppy hands. He was good at holding toys which fitted into the palm of his hand, but he was not good at picking things up with his fingers—perhaps because most of the toys he gravitated towards tended to be of the ball or rattle variety, and were no challenge to him. We started to experiment. A large plastic peg man presented no problem. He placed his palm over the top of its head, curled his fingers round its body and could manipulate it quite efficiently. We moved on to chunky wooden peg men, about the diameter of a broomstick (made by Escor Toys, address on p. 8). These were a little more problematical. In order to place them upright in the holes made for them in the bus that formed part of the toy, (see p. 104) he had to grasp them round the neck. Although he often dropped a man, he wanted to fill the bus with passengers, so persevered until it was full. Over the weeks ahead, we were able to offer him toys with smaller peg men. As he grew older and more proficient, we made him a 'one off' posting box from a tin with a polythene lid, similar to the one described on p. 76. We cut a slit in the lid and gave him some very large buttons to post inside. These needed to be picked up carefully, and angled correctly. Of course, they made a satisfying clatter when they dropped into the tin.

TOYS TO ENCOURAGE A PINCHING MOVEMENT

A Colour Peg Tin

Long-lasting

This toy makes use of old-fashioned wooden dolly pegs. These have a neatly turned head, a body and two legs, which normally straddle the washing on the line. Peg tins have been around for many years and are often seen in classrooms. Here they are used for hand-eye co-ordination and colour matching, but they are also excellent for practising a pinching movement. The toy is made from a square biscuit tin. Each side is painted a different colour and a collection of matching dolly pegs

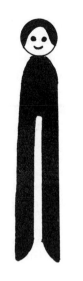

lie in the bottom. Toddlers love the clatter the pegs make as they are stirred around in the tin. Before long they learn to place them on the rim of the tin, unwittingly using their pincer grip and, in the process, practising their hand-eye co-ordination too! Older ones use the tin as intended and slot the pegs over the sides which match them in colour. As an added bonus the toy makes its own container.

Materials
- A deep, square biscuit tin.
- Dolly pegs—say a packet of thirty six.
- Humbrol enamel in four colours.
- Black, waterproof fibre-tipped pen.
- Polyurethane varnish.
- A cardboard carton—useful for holding the pegs while they dry.

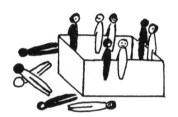

Method
Paint one side of the tin, inside and out. While you wait for the paint to dry, start on the peg men. With the fibre-tipped pen, draw a face on each—two dots for eyes and a smiley mouth. Divide the pegs into four sets. On one set paint hats and bodies to match the finished side of the tin. Perch the pegs on the side of the carton to dry. Using the remaining three colours, paint the other sides and their sets of peg men. When all the pegs are dry, dip the heads in polyurethane varnish (to prevent the faces from being rubbed off with much handling) and perch them back on the carton. Brush any excess varnish over their bodies and legs to prevent 'runs'.

Note
Over the years the metal used to make biscuit tins has become thinner. Sometimes, with rough use, the seams can split apart. If the tin is used by a group, check it frequently for sharp edges or avoid the problem by substituting four coffee tins (or similar) with turned lips and polythene lids. Paint each tin and its collection of pegs a different colour. Make circular holes in the lids, and the toy can double up as a set of simple one-hole posting boxes.

A Peg Bus

Long-lasting

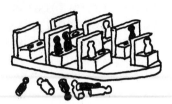

The bus, as in the illustration, also uses dolly pegs, but now they are truncated. Simply saw off the 'legs' of the peg and you are left with a little peg man about 4 cm (1½") tall. The toy is meant to represent the school minibus. It has no wheels! This is on purpose. The bus keeps steady, while a child locates the passengers in their holes and, of course, it simplifies the construction.

Materials
● Suitable wood for the base, seats and seat backs.
● Truncated dolly pegs—as many as you need, plus a few spares.
● Paint for the peg men—in several colours, if you want to use them for colour matching (two the same on one seat).
● Sandpaper.
● Polyurethane varnish for overall protection.

Method
Decide on the proportions of your toy. How many seats? Will they be arranged in pairs, like mine, or would a single line of seats be more appropriate for the child in question? Cut your peg men from dolly pegs. Sketch out a plan of the bus, remembering that the size of the seats is dependent on the girth of the peg men. Cut a suitable piece of thick ply or MDF (Medium Density Fibreboard) to be the base. Its shape is roughly like an iron and the length of mine from front to back about 30 cm (12"). The seats need to be about 7½ cm (3") × 4 cm (1½") on the top to allow for two peg men to sit side by side. The height of the seat from the floor should be about 3 cm (1¼").Drill two holes in each seat, slightly larger than the peg men, and deep enough for them to fit in without wobbling about. Add a plywood back to each seat. This adds a touch of realism and makes it easier for a child to guide a peg man into his hole. (He can't overshoot!) Countersink, screw and glue the backs to the seats. Countersink, screw and glue the seats to the bus. Paint the peg men. In my version, the driver sits up front in a white coat and the passengers in pairs, according to the colour of their clothes, fill up the bus behind him (or her).

The peg bus lends itself to story telling. Two peg children sitting side by side can have a conversation, or even fall out with each other. A peg child sitting behind might act as a peacemaker!

A Colour Peg Board

Long-lasting

Dolly peg men are also used to make this toy. It does not have such opportunities for imaginative play as the bus above, but it is useful as an extra colour-matching toy and certainly gives plenty of practice in putting pegs in holes. It had many fans among the children with learning difficulties and minor hand-function problems who played with the prototype. For economy, a fairly large piece of chip-board was used for the base, which measured 24 cm (9") × 32 cm (12"). This was marked out into 8 cm (3") squares. A hole was drilled in the centre of all the twelve squares, ready to receive a peg man. Then each square and its man was painted a different colour. The task for the children was to place each round peg in the appropriate round hole.

SPRING-LOADED CLOTHES PEGS

For many children, playing with Mum's peg bag is one of the delights of wash day. They will clip the pegs end-to-end to make a long line, or will form them into a zigzag. They may even clip them to their noses or other ridiculous places. This play does not help wash day along, but it does wonders for the children's 'pinching action'!

Now for some popular toys which also provide therapy through play.

Clothes Peg Puppets

Quick

Turn a clothes peg sideways on and pinch the end. Immediately the peg appears to be opening its mouth! The simple little puppets which follow make use of this movement. Basically, they are just circles of reasonably sturdy cardboard glued to a *wooden* peg. Three examples are illustrated, but once you have the idea, no end of characters can be created . . . all capable of talking to each other in profile.

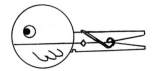

The Fish

Begin with a circle of thin card, say 6 cm (2¼") in diameter. If you make it much larger, it will be too heavy to stick to the average clothes peg. Colour the fish. Cut it in two, making the bottom jaw smaller than the upper. Stick both pieces to the peg, just in front of the spring, making sure they close together properly. Use a strong glue (e.g. U-Hu) and hold the pieces in place until it dries. The basic fish can be embellished with fins and a small tail either cut out with the circle or added afterwards. Experiment!

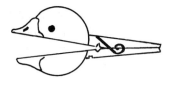

The Duck

This is based on the same circular shape, but has a bill added to the circle before cutting out. If you are teaching your child the rhyme about the five little ducks who went swimming one day (p. 42), this puppet makes a *quick* Mother Duck. It is also useful if you sing 'Old Macdonald Had a Farm'. Other animal heads can be made on the same principle.

The Alligator

Another variation on the theme, but this time the jaws are lengthened and they are separated by a zigzag cut to represent the fierce teeth.

A Plastic Milk Bottle Monster

Long-lasting

Anne Smith,
Paediatric
Occupational
Therapist

This monster comes from the realms of fantasy. It is chubby and tough. With its clothes peg 'spines' clipped in place, it could be a dinosaur, or even an exotic fish! The screw top to the milk bottle makes the mouth. The top—and possibly the sides—have cardboard protuberances (called 'fins' for want of a better word) to which the pegs can be clipped. Putting them on and taking them off will require plenty of 'pinching', and putting them away inside the bottle at the end of the session is another way to practise 'posting'!

Materials
- A plastic milk bottle.
- Plenty of spring-loaded clothes pegs, say a dozen.
- A small amount of cardboard, such as a cereal packet.

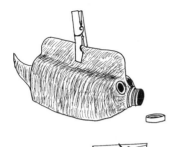

- Newspaper and paste for the papier mâché coating. For details, see p. 3.
- Sellotape.
- Paint. Acrylic is best, but poster or powder paint will do.
- Polyurethane varnish for protection and to make the toy wipeable.

Method

Wash out the milk bottle thoroughly. To make a fin, cut a strip of cardboard about 15 cm (6") wide and as long as the milk bottle. Fold it in half along its length and splay out the bottom edges. Glue the centre part of the fin together. It should be about 5 cm (2") deep, so that the clothes pegs will clip to it properly. Round off its corners. Fit it to the bottle, keeping it in place with Sellotape. Anne makes fins for the sides too. In my version, I added a tail! You may have your own ideas. Now cover the whole creature (except the mouth of course) with papier mâché. Try to keep the fins a good shape. If you use too much paste, you will find they tend to become floppy. If you are too generous with the layers of paper, the pegs will not clip on well, but make sure the places where they join the bottle are well covered. When the paste is dry, paint the monster. Give it prominent eyes and a coat of mottled green and brown ... or what you will. When the paint is dry, protect it with a coat of polyurethane varnish and when that is dry, store the pegs inside, and the monster is ready for play.

MORE TOYS TO PINCH

A Marble Maze

Long-lasting

This is a toy that is easy to adapt to individual needs. It consists of two layers of cloth stitched together in such a way that channels are formed. The challenge for the child is to squeeze a marble through the channels so that it will travel from point A to point B. By making the arrangement of the channels simple (perhaps just a short spiral) or more complicated with blind alleys here and there, as in a real maze, the toy can be made appropriate to the ability of the child. Large marbles can

107

be pinched through wide channels, or small beads coaxed through narrow ones. As usual the choice is yours.

Materials

- Scrap paper for planning your maze.
- Fabric for the cloth sandwich. Unbleached calico is ideal—perhaps used with gingham, which is already printed in squares and gives instant guide lines for the channels.
- Some transparent fabric for 'windows' at the start and finish points, e.g. net curtaining. Alternatively, the whole of the top layer of the cloth sandwich can

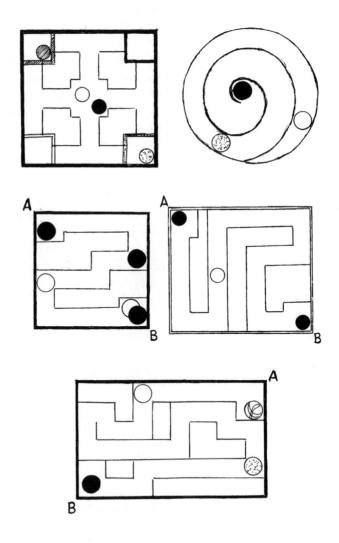

be made of net and the child can then *see* the progress of the marble along the channel.

- A marble (maybe more than one) or bead(s).
- Bias binding—optional, but it makes a colourful and neat frame to the toy. A sewing machine with a zigzag stitch is useful and time-saving, but not essential. The channels can be made by hand, using a small running stitch.

Method

First plan your maze on paper. You will need to draw it to scale, but first make sure a marble (or bead) will go through the channels with just the right amount of effort. If the channel is too narrow, the marble will stick. If it is too wide, the marble will simply roll through without any need to 'pinch'. As a rough estimate, the channels need to be just over one and a half times the diameter of the marble. Trial and error is the only safe way to check this. Make some mock channels on two layers of scrap material and try them for size. (I have a ruler which is just the right width for this job. It saves me a lot of accurate measuring!) Having decided on the width of your channels, you can now draw your maze design to scale. Cut out the top and bottom layers of the maze. In pencil, transfer your design to the underside of the *bottom* layer of the cloth sandwich. (The pencil lines are useful later as a sewing guide.) Now attend to the *top* layer. If you are *not* using net curtaining throughout, cut out the beginning and end windows and replace them with net to prevent the marble from escaping! Zigzag round the edges of the windows to keep the net in place. Pin the top and bottom layers together. Turn them over so that the bottom is uppermost. Set your machine to the narrowest and closest zigzag. Follow your pencil marks and stitch both layers together to form the channels. Stitch bias binding (or use a wider zigzag stitch) to close up the outside edges. *Remember to put in the marble* before you complete this job!

Apart from being an excellent toy for encouraging the use of finger tips and pinching, this simple puzzle makes a welcome travelling companion for children on a long journey, or even a daily trip on the school bus. As already mentioned, it can be made in a variety of designs. It is washable, unswallowable, virtually inde-structible and easy to send by post. What more could you want?

Pinchums

Long-lasting

These delightful little talking heads originated, I think, in the USA. They are worked in wool over plastic canvas. Basically, each one is made from three squares. The directions are given for the 'Mother Duck', which plays an important role in the rhyme on p. 42, but the principle is easy to adapt for other animal heads, e.g. a frog with bulbous eyes added, a fox with felt pointed ears or a badger with its distinc-tive white head stripes. You will see from the diagram that when the three pieces are assembled, the back of the head acts as a spring, keeping the mouth closed. Pinch the cheeks at the appropriate moment and the puppet opens its bill to say 'Quack' on cue ... (or whatever sound is appropriate to a badger etc!) Once you have made your first one, you may think of many more ways of using the pattern.

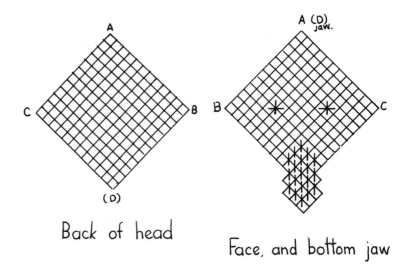

Back of head

Face, and bottom jaw

Materials
- Seven–mesh plastic canvas—from a craft shop or by mail order (p. 7).
- Wool—tapestry or DK (double knitting). For the duck, white for most of the head, yellow for the bill and

mouth, black for the eyes. Other animals as appropriate.

● A tapestry needle. This has a large eye and a blunt point.

Method

Start by cutting out the back of the head. This is the simplest shape, just a square. Make it 13 bars each way, (12 holes). Now for the face and bottom jaw, as in the diagram. These are based on the same square, but a bill is added. I find it helpful to run a tacking stitch from point A to the tip of the bill. I delay cutting out the bill until I am certain these two points will line up. If you snip off an extra bar by accident, the bill will be too narrow. Count the bars carefully! Complete the cutting out. Next we come to the stitching. Begin with the back of the head. Cover it with cross stitch or tent stitch. If the canvas shows through, use the wool double. Then cover the face, stitching the bill in yellow. Add the eyes *now* as it is impossible to stitch them on once the head is assembled. Cover the bottom jaw, in the same way, but omitting the eyes of course! Finally, oversew the pieces together as in the diagram, i.e. join AB on the face to AB on the back of the head, and AC to AC. Make extra stitches at A to make sure the point of the canvas is covered. Oversew the bottom jaw to the back of the head by joining DB to DB and DC to DC. In yellow, oversew all the way round the duck's bill to cover the exposed edge of canvas.

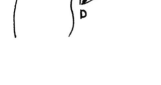

A Button Tapper

Quick

Robert Race,
Maker of Automata
and Adult Toys

I learnt how to make this delightful little toy when attending one of Robert's toymaking courses. It can be assembled very quickly from a plastic lid and a large button, with a rubber band to provide the action. Its life is not endless but, while it survives, it is superb for practising the pinching action, and gives great pleasure to the children.

Materials

● A lid for the top of the toy. This can be one from a plastic milk bottle, or from a jar of Marmite, Bovril, etc.

● An elastic band.

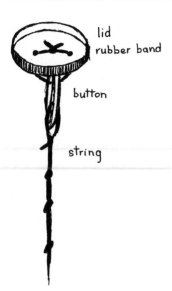

lid
rubber band

button

string

- A coat button with holes large enough to accept the (cut) elastic band.
- A length of string—say a bit less than a metre (yard) and thin enough to go through a hole in the button.
- An awl or any spiked tool to make holes. (For adult use.)

Method
Make two holes in the lid. Cut the band and thread it through a hole in the button. Hold the lid upside down. Thread the loose ends of elastic up through the two holes in the lid. Tie the ends together firmly, making *sure* the rim of the button is pulled against the lid. Make knots at regular intervals all down the string. Thread one end through the button (the opposite hole to the one with the band through it) and tie it on firmly.

Now for the action. Hold the lid with one hand and, with the other, gently pinch the string. As you slide your thumb and finger down the string, every time you reach a knot the button will pull away from the lid. As you pass the knot, the button will snap back against it. Perform this sliding action speedily and you will make the sound of a heavy shower on a tin roof or a woodpecker at work! Do it more slowly and you can imagine a clock ticking. I guess you find this quite soothing and therapeutic. Be unselfish and now let your child have a go!

Pointing

ISOLATING ONE FINGER

At a meeting of our Active Group, (see p. x) someone asked if we could think up some ways of helping a child to isolate one finger, i.e. *point*! It seems this is quite a common problem. We began a 'brainstorming session' and offered various *instant* suggestions which may be helpful to anyone playing with a child who has this problem.

With one finger . . .

- Trace along a line on the carpet, tablecloth, pattern on the furniture.
- Draw in the steam on the window pane.
- Prod into a lump of Playdough (recipes pp. 99/100).
- Play a game of 'Put your finger on your . . .' nose, ear, tongue, etc.
- Play a keyboard instrument.
- Play a metal xylophone with a thimble on the finger.
- Use Touch and Play music buttons from the Craft Depot, (p. 7). These must be mounted on a base, such as a fairly large square of thick card, or it is possible to activate them by squeezing!
- Slide a Smartie top or a button with a lip around a tray or the table top. Have races.
- Use the dicky bird finger puppets etc. on p. 40.

One Hole Finger Puppets

Very quick

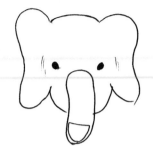

Make one-hole finger puppets from cardboard, such as the elephant illustrated. Invent your own characters.

If you are temporarily at a loss for ideas, why not try a wiggly worm? This is the simplest of all one finger puppets and makes a good 'prop' if you want to introduce your child to Wiggly Woo. All you need is an irregular shape cut-out of card, (about the size of a saucer) to hide your hand. Colour one side brown to represent the soil, and make a hole in the centre for a finger to poke through. Now make a smaller shape for the child, colour it brown and make a finger hole in the centre as before. With the 'soil' resting on your fists and fingers in the holes you are both ready for the rhyme about Wiggly Woo!

There's a worm at the bottom of my garden,
And his name is Wiggly Woo.
There's a worm at the bottom of my garden,
Oh dear! What shall I do?
He wiggles all night and he wiggles all day.
The people all look round and say
'There's a worm at the bottom of your garden,
And his name is Wiggly Woo!'

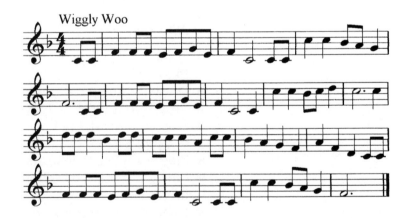

Nosy Rosie

Quick

Make a 'Nosy Rosie' puppet from a polystyrene drinking cup. This idea comes from an American book, '1–2–3 Puppets' written by Jean Warren. Jean cuts a nose hole in the side of the cup for a finger to poke through, (Nosy Rosie's nose!), adds features with felt pens and a few

114

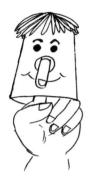

wisps of wool for hair, glued to the bottom of the cup—now the top of the head. Then Nosy Rosie can roam the room sniffing at whatever takes her fancy. This little ditty is sung to the tune of 'Here we go round the mulberry bush':

Here comes old Nosy Rosie,
Nosy Rosie, Nosy Rosie,
Here comes old Nosy Rosie,
Sniff, sniff, sniffing flowers (or what you will).

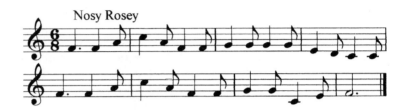

Nosy Rosey

115

Using both hands

Persuading a child to use a 'lazy' hand when the other is so much more efficient can be an uphill task. If the problem is ignored, it will not go away but, if too much fuss is made, the child is likely to set up a resistance which is hard to break. In the course of the usual busy day, it is difficult to think up surreptitious ways of involving the use of both hands, but incidental therapy through play is well worth considering. Here are some simple ideas to fall back on and, if successful, they may well lead on to others thought up by you.

Rhymes and Finger Plays

Instant

For young children, some rhymes and jingles can come in handy, particularly those which involve clapping. Perhaps the most obvious one is 'Pat-a-Cake', and there are others among the 'Rhymes for Finger Play', p. 35. Here are two more rhymes that use a winding movement, one hand tumbling over the other.

116

Wind the bobbin up
  Wind the bobbin up, wind the bobbin up,
  (*suit the actions to the words*)
  Pull . . ., pull . . ., clap, clap, clap,
  (*pull sideways and clap loudly*)
  Wind the bobbin up, wind the bobbin up,
  Pull . . ., pull . . ., clap, clap, clap.
  Point to the ceiling, point to the door,
  Point to the window, point to the floor,
  Put your hands together, one, two, three,
  (*clap three times*)
  Put your hands upon your knee.

Roly poly up
Say this one quite slowly so that there is plenty of
winding movement.

  Roly poly up, up, up
  (*raise your arms as your hands rotate around each
  other*)
  Roly poly down, down down,
  (*lower them*)
  Roly poly clap, clap, clap,
  Put your hands behind your back.
  (*wiggle your fingers as you do this.*)

SOME ACTIVITIES AND TOYS

- Play a game of 'throw and catch' using a large, light
  object like a beach ball or a scatter cushion.
- Make an opportunity for the child to carry something
  (unspillable and unbreakable) on a tray.
- Helping around the house can provide many opportunities for using both hands—using a dustpan and
  brush for one.
- Provide a low washing line and let the child help to
  hang out the washing.
- A long broom or a squeezy mop needs both hands to
  guide it successfully, and the same can be said for a
  rake to collect up the Autumn leaves.
- A wheelbarrow will not work unless both hands
  grasp the handles.

- Threading is an activity which involves both hands, and it has a section all to itself. 'Proper' threading may be too difficult for many children, but there are other ways of using the threading action which may be possible and appealing. For example, threading unwanted keys onto a large treasury tag kept Alice amused for a considerable time. Treasury tags are lengths of cord with metal tags at both ends. They come in an assortment of sizes and are available at all large stationers.

- Peter was persuaded to lift up his 'lazy' hand and wave it about when it was slipped inside a tube cut from an old washing-up liquid bottle. With his able hand he could slide the tube down his arm so that his hand would pop out of the top—like a game of 'Peep-Bo'. This was even more successful when a face was painted on his fist (using face paints).He found this simple game hilarious!

- Many percussion instruments require the use of both hands, and the joy of making a loud noise can be very motivating. The following are worth a try—cymbals, a tambourine, a pair of maraccas or bongo drums.

Now for some *Quick* ideas.

Making a Woolly Ball or a Woolly Doll

These two activities encourage the child to make use of a winding movement and both can lead on to further play. The ball, of course, can be used for throwing and catching, and the dolls make good occupants for the dolls' house, passengers in a train, etc. They are not suitable for children who may get their fingers caught between the strands of wool.

Directions for making the woolly ball are on p. 79.

You may already be familiar with woolly dolls from memories of your own childhood. If so, you will need no help from me! If the idea is new to you, I suggest you make a doll yourself, then show your child how to do it. Your help will be needed when it comes to the binding and tying part. Start by making a small hank for the arms by grouping three fingers together and winding the wool over them about ten times.(The thickness of the wool will be the deciding factor.) Carefully slip the wool off your fingers and bind round and tie both ends

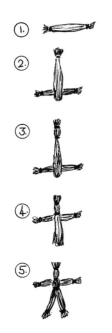

of the hank to make the wrists, as in illustration (1). Lay the hank aside while you make a larger and fatter hank to be the rest of the doll. Separate out all your fingers on one hand and wind over them as before. (Wind round about twenty times.) Pick up the arms and slide them into the 'body' hank before you ease it off your fingers. (If you don't put the arms in at this stage, the loops of wool that make up the 'body' hank can get out of order, and it is then more difficult to insert the arms into it.) Bind and tie the 'body' hank very near the top (2). The loops at the top will be cut later to make the hair. A little lower down, bind and tie again to make the face and neck (3). Slide the arms up, tight against the neck. Make sure they are of equal length each side of the body and bind and tie them in place (4). Separate out the rest of the hank to make the legs. Bind and tie round each ankle (5). Cut the loops of wool at the top of the doll to represent hair and add wool features if you wish.

A Marble Maze on a Tray

The useful art of learning to carry a tray can easily be developed into an interesting game. Provide a ball—tennis perhaps?—or a marble, large or small, to be directed through a maze by the simple means of skilfully tipping the tray, this way and that. Start with an old tea tray, or a large baking tray. Line the bottom with thick paper or thin card anchoring it down with double-sided Sellotape. Make the walls of the maze with thick string. First plan the route in pencil, making sure the walls are the right distance apart for the ball or marble to roll easily between them. (The patterns for the cloth mazes on p. 108 may give you inspiration.) Squirt or paint a line of PVA glue over the pencil lines and press the string onto the glue. Leave to dry.

Thread a 'Clanky'

This simple pull-along toy must be made by the child. It is just a collection of unwanted, unbreakable, thread-able objects—preferably metal ones which will make a noise when pulled along such as a dented saucepan lid (with a handle, not a knob), or an old (chipped?) tin mug, and you might even provide an old sandal perhaps, or a short cardboard tube . . . in fact, any scrap object with a hole or slot in it that can be threaded. The

119

threader is a length of thick string with the end stiffened (for easy manipulation). This can be done by doubling it over and binding it with thin string or wool, or by dipping the end in PVA glue, rolling it into a point and leaving it to dry. Once the objects have been threaded onto the string, the child can have the joy of towing them triumphantly at top speed down the concrete garden path!

Giant Building Bricks

Jane was persuaded, inadvertently, to use her 'lazy' hand when her mother and I made her and her little friend a set of oversize building bricks. A plea to the neighbours soon provided a collection of sturdy washing powder boxes. These were stuffed with crunched-up newspaper to make them even stronger, and the openings sealed with plastic tape. With this basic material, the girls could build little shelters for their dolls, walls for hiding behind, roadways for walking along, etc. Less sturdy, hollow cardboard boxes were added to the collection, and could be stacked to make a tower, or nested one inside another. They could also be turned this way or that to become a car, or boat, to sit in, or tortoise shell to be worn on the back! When nearing the end of their life, they could be jumped on and flattened before taking them to their final resting place—the recycling bin.

A Visi-Tube

A simple and unusual toy to encourage the use of both hands evolved because of a need. James could just about hold things (reluctantly) with one hand, but naturally preferred to use the other more able one whenever possible. Our challenge was to try to persuade him to change his habits! Many of the ideas above were useful, but he made his best efforts when provided with a large Visi-Tube. This was just a length of wide transparent polythene tubing about the diameter of a garden hose. One end was blocked off with a cork, pushed well inside the tube so that it could only be extracted with a corkscrew. Small beads and the smallest sized marbles were put in the tube before the open end was blocked off with another cork. The idea was to grasp the tube at both ends then tip the contents from one end to the other. James found this entrancing.

He loved the noise the contents made as they slid down the tube and the toy was also visually interesting. As a further development, we blocked off a section of the tube with masking tape so that the contents could be hidden behind it.

I made a similar tube for another, very verbal, child. She liked me to make up little stories concerning the contents. One day the beads and marbles might be some children scuttling to hide behind the masked-off area taking shelter from the rain. Another time, the contents might be a train going through a tunnel, and having to stop just outside to allow the passengers to alight. All 'therapy without tears'!

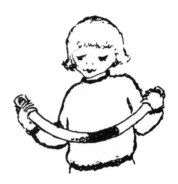

Threading

Threading is a peaceful play activity with many a useful spin-off. It requires the use of both hands as well as hand-eye co-ordination. It can also help to develop other skills such as colour matching, sorting, grading and sequencing. Leaving aside all these worthy attributes, most children at some stage in their lives really *enjoy* threading beads!

First of all, the action of poking the threader through the hole must be learnt.

- In an Australian toy library they really start from scratch by showing the children how to thread large hair curlers onto a length of plastic pipe.
- At Lekotek Korea, they use blocks of wood with holes bored through them and a piece of dowel to be the threader.
- At some toy libraries in the UK, the children thread plastic rings, cut from a washing-up liquid bottle, over their arms like bangles.

Threading toys are, of course, available from toy shops, but here is an excellent one you can make yourself.

The Bee in a Tree

Long-lasting

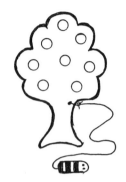

This delightful threading toy first appeared in the 'Making Toys' programme televised by the BBC. Its designer, David Chisnell, created a plywood tree shape, which had several holes drilled in the leafy part. One end of a length of cord was tied to the tree trunk, and the other was attached to a short length of dowel which represented the busy bee. The bee could 'fly' in and out of the holes until all the string was used up.

Materials
- For the tree, either an old table tennis bat with the rubber face removed, or a small piece of good quality ply, 5 mm or 7 mm,
- About 5 cm (2") of dowel for the bee, or you could use a long, fat macramé bead.
- A length of thin cord for attaching the bee to the tree say 20–30 cm (8–12") or longer, depending on how far the child in question can stretch. Blind cord is best. This will not kink.
- A dab of strong adhesive (such as a wood glue or Evostick) and a matchstick (for fixing the cord in the hole in the bee).
- Sandpaper.
- Paint, and polyurethane varnish for protection.

You will also need a fret saw or electric jig saw, a large drill for the holes for the bee to fly through, and a small drill to make the hole for inserting the cord in the rear end of the bee.

Method
Draw a tree shape on the plywood as suggested in the illustration. The broadening out of the tree trunk makes it easier to grasp. Cut out the tree. Drill holes at intervals in the leafy part. Drill a small hole in the trunk for the threading cord. Clean up all the rough edges with sandpaper. Round off the face end of the dowel bee (with sandpaper) and drill a small hole in its other end to take the threading cord. Paint both sides of the tree green, with a brown trunk. Paint the bee yellow with black stripes and give it a face. Protect all the paint with two coats of polyurethane varnish. Tie one end of the cord to the tree trunk. Squirt some glue into the hole in

123

the bee and poke in the other end of the cord. A needle is helpful to feed it in. Wedge it firmly in place with a small piece of matchstick coated with adhesive.

THREADING BEADS

Homemade beads for children with poor hand control

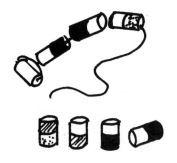

Children who find threading very difficult may get on better if they have large beads with almost unmissable holes in the centre, and a threader they can grasp easily. It is worthwhile trying to meet these two requirements, for a child who can thread a bead may also be able, in time, to do up a button. With a little effort, a bead with a virtually unmissable hole can be made from the cardboard tubes found in the centres of paper towel rolls. Each tube will cut into about four beads. It does not matter if they are different sizes. In their raw state they are much too floppy and may tend to become unwrapped. Papier mâché has already been used to strengthen toys in this book, and it can come to the rescue again here (see p. 3). Cover each card bead with enough layers to make it uncrushable (still keeping the large hole in the middle). Finish off with a layer of white paper or a coat of white paint, and decorate to your own artistic satisfaction. Protect your works of art with polyurethane varnish. Make a threader from a length of dowel. This should be at least twice as long as the largest bead so that, when one is threaded onto it, the dowel will protrude and can be grasped by the child's free hand. Round off the threading end. Drill a small hole in the other, and glue in the threading string, wedging it in place with a slither of matchstick, as for the Bee in a Tree above. Remember to tie a 'stopper' on the end of the string to prevent the beads from dropping off.

Note
If a child has unco-ordinated movements and is likely to hit his face with a long threader, this one is not for him. See suggested threaders opposite and on p.122.

Making a necklace

It takes a steady hand to hold a bead in position and aim a threader through the hole in the middle. Avoid the frustration (and possible bad temper) that can happen if beads roll out of reach, or the threader will not go through the hole easily. Here are some tips to consider.

- Provide a container for the beads. A plastic cereal bowl is ideal. If keeping it upright or in one place is a problem, fix it to the table with a blob of Blu-tac, or a loop of masking tape.
- Put the bowl on a tray with a lip and the chances of beads escaping is reduced even more.
- Brightly-coloured wooden beads can be bought at most toy shops. For children who find threading difficult, choose square ones. These are easier to hold between finger and thumb and will not roll away.
- Attractive adult beads which appeal to older children can sometimes be bought cheaply at car boot sales, charity shops, etc.
- Make sure the threader will go right through the bead and out the other side. Sometimes a round shoelace will do the job, but large beads may need a special threader with a long tag available from educational suppliers. Nearer to hand is the polypropylene clothes line—the thin one without a wire core, used for whirly lines. This goes through the large holes in wooden beads very successfully, and is stiff enough to come well out of the hole for easy grasping and pulling through.
- Jewellers sell nylon threaders with a stiff wire end. These are excellent for children who wish to thread small beads.

Making your own paper beads

Homemade paper beads have been around for so long that they might even be considered traditional toys. They are made by rolling up strips of paper. All you need is a knitting needle, (the larger the size, the bigger the hole in the middle will be), a strip of paper, some PVA adhesive, (diluted a little for economy and easier spreading)—or flour and water paste, p.5 and some acrylic or poster paint, or felt pens, for decorating the finished beads.

Use a non-shiny white paper such as ceiling lining paper or flat (not embossed) wallpaper. If you use wallpaper, the beads will be chunkier and you will need a shorter strip. If you use newspaper, the finished beads will need a coat of white paint to mask the newsprint before they can be decorated.

Against the edge of the table, or a ruler, tear the paper into strips say 24 cm × 5 cm (10" × 2"). Take one strip and start to wind it round the knitting needle until the end is tucked in. Then paste the rest of the strip and continue to wind it tightly round the needle to form a cylinder. Slide this off the needle and put it to one side to dry. It is best to wind near the tip of the needle so that the bead will slip off easily. Wipe the needle before making the next bead in case any adhesive has been left behind. When you have become skilful in rolling these beads, you might try larger or smaller ones or even give them a rounded shape by using strips of paper that taper off like a pennant. Once the adhesive is dry, the beads can be decorated.

Buttons

The skills needed to poke a button through a hole are quite considerable. Anyone who has struggled to teach a small child to master the art before her first day at school—that major leap towards independence—will have realised that the task is far from simple. The button must be held by its rim and guided, end on, through a tiny slot, then grasped by the other hand and pulled completely through until it lies flat on the surface of the garment. Not easy! Children with minor hand-function problems may happily achieve this self-help skill if the process is broken down for them. Once a child has learnt to pinch, a first stage may be just learning to angle the buttons by posting them through a slot in the lid of a tin (p. 102). When it comes to the serious business of doing up (or undoing) buttons on clothes, begin with one large button on a coat laid flat on the table, that the child can *see*. At first let her poke the button through the hole, then finish off the job by pulling it through for her. When she can manage the whole process on her own, she might progress to the bottom button of a coat worn by you. The next stage is the bottom button of her own coat. Once the button is safely through the hole, it should also be undone. This also helps the child learn to undress. If left to her own devices, she is likely to try to undo buttons by clutching at the edges of her garment and ripping them apart in the hope that the button will escape from its hole. Usual result—a ripped off button!

As the child's skill increases and coat buttons can be managed, move on to slightly smaller ones. With a row of buttons, say on a cardigan, again begin at the bottom. This way each button should go through the correct hole and not the one next to it.

Now for a variety of ideas designed to foster the skill of 'buttoning' through play.

A Buttoning Jar

Very quick

Nora Lack,
Paediatric
Occupational
Therapist

This toy is very popular with Nora's young patients. They happily slot squares of felt over a button on the end of a length of cord for the joy of seeing their 'garland' grow longer and longer. On the practical side, the toy is cheap, easy and quick to make, and at the end of the 'Buttoning Session' it makes its own container.

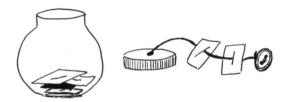

Materials
- A plastic food jar with a screwtop lid.
- A length of string or cord—say 40 cm (16").
- A large button.
- Plenty of small felt squares, Say 8 cm (3"). Nora buys hers ready cut from a craft shop.

Method
Punch a hole in the centre of the lid. Poke one end of the cord through it. Tie a large knot on the underside to prevent it from pulling out. Tie the button to the other end. You may need to separate the strands of the cord and tie them together on the top of the button. Cut slots in all the squares of felt. These must be large enough for

the button to go through easily, but they will stretch with use, so take care not to make the slots too generous. Put most of the felt squares in the jar, but keep a few in reserve as replacements for any that go astray, become grubby, misshapen or torn with much use. Now the child can dive in the jar and 'buttoning' can begin. At the end of the session, the squares should be removed from the string and replaced in the jar before screwing on the lid. This gives useful practice in that other skill—'unbuttoning'!

Button Chains

Quick

An Idea from
Canberra Toy Library,
Australia

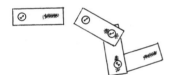

Children love to make daisy chains Here the daisies are represented by pieces of felt. A button is sewn to one end of each piece and a corresponding slot cut in the other end.

Make each piece say 4 × 15 cm (1½ × 6") All the buttons (and the slots) should be roughly the same size.

For a *long-lasting* button chain, back the felt pieces with another fabric. Lycra is ideal. It stretches, but it does not fray, and a single row of running stitches round the edges of each rectangle is all that is necessary. (Alternatively, use cotton and attach the felt to it by zigzagging round the edge.) I make light of this job by sticking the felt piece to the unmeasured piece of lycra with Pritt Stick, stitch around the edges, then cut out the new rectangle of felt backed with lycra. I make strong, stitched buttonholes as opposed to slits, and attach the buttons with little 'stalks', so that they are easier to twist and poke through. The result is a tough toy which will stand much pulling and tweaking.

Note
To make a button 'stalk', place two matchsticks under the button, between it and the felt. These act as a spacer. Sew the button on firmly, remove the matchsticks, twist the button thread several times round the underside of the button and fasten off securely.

Button Trainers

Long-lasting

I made a series of these for a group of children with learning difficulties and mild hand-function problems. The idea was to give the children practice in handling buttons not attached to their clothes. Using a button trainer, they could see what they were doing and could handle the buttons at a convenient distance from their bodies.

Stage one was like a two-page rag book. With the spine of the book on the left, two large buttonholes were made in the top page and corresponding buttons sewn to the bottom one. The task was to poke the buttons through the holes so that they sat on the top of the book. The children could soon manage this, so the next stage was to make another two-page book, but this time the number of buttons was increased to four. They were meant to represent flowers, so the buttonholes on the top page were embellished with stalks and leaves. When the buttons were in place, we had a miniature garden. There was a limit to the number of buttons that could be used with the book format. More than six, and it was difficult to handle those sewn near to the spine.

Stage three solved the problem. This trainer was circular, with buttons and holes positioned round the edge so that all could be reached easily. I used a dinner plate as a template and cut two circles of fabric to be the top and bottom of the trainer—the former for the button holes and the latter for the buttons. To avoid raw edges and to give the fabric extra strength, both circles were lined. Then they were pinned together at the edges. Using a saucer as a template, I drew round it in the centre of the top circle. The pencil mark acted as a sewing guide as I stitched the circles together. With the pins removed, the final stage was to sew attractive buttons to the bottom circle and make appropriate buttonholes in the top one. All the buttons were now easy to manipulate.

This button trainer was all very well in its way, but it did not hold the children's interest for long. Remembering its plate-like origins, I decided to add some food! In an odd moment, using some offcuts of thin ply, I cut out the shapes of a fried egg, sausages, mushrooms and tomatoes and painted them. By drilling two small holes in the centre of each, they became buttonlike and could be attached to a pair of fabric circles as above. Now, using the same movements as those needed to do up a button, a full English breakfast could be threaded through the buttonholes made to receive all the different-sized food shapes. This toy was *funny* and had instant appeal for the group in question.

A Car Button Trainer

Long-lasting

At the toy library we have an ongoing need for a variety of button trainers. This one, based on the simple ones above is a popular favourite. It is also like a two-page book. The pages are made from calico. On the top page is appliqued a picture of a child sitting in a car, waiting for the lights to change. The picture is unfinished. There are buttonholes to receive the wheels, the steering wheel and the traffic lights. The buttons to make up these essential elements are stitched to the bottom page. Even reluctant 'buttoners' need no coaxing to finish off the picture.

A Button Snake

Long-lasting

This peculiar reptile is just a series of cloth segments, reducing in size from head to tail, each buttoning to the one in front. There is an element of 'matching' involved. The buttons are arranged in pairs and are chosen for their interesting shapes or colours. In play, the snake is dismembered and all its segments are jumbled up. The child finds the head, then looks for the matching button on the next segment. These segments are buttoned together. The child notices a new button and searches for its twin on the next segment . . . and so on until the tail is reached.

Materials
- Pairs of buttons—the number and size according to the ability of the children.
- Fabric, for top pieces and linings, e.g. cotton, calico.
- Button thread.
- Card—for making the templates.
- Scraps of black and white felt or embroidery thread for the eyes.

Method

Make card templates for all the segments. The largest for the head and first segment, should be about 10 × 14 cm (4 × 5½"). The next segment is about 1½ cm (½") narrower, and so on all down the line. To make the top pieces and linings, put the templates on the wrong side of the fabric and draw round them. Cut outside the pencil lines. They come in handy later as a stitching guide. Round off the head and tail. Lay all the pieces out in front of you—top pieces, linings and pairs of buttons. Beginning with the pieces for the head, put right sides

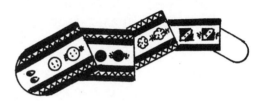

together and pin. Following the pencil line, stitch most of the way round. Remove the pins and turn right side out. Close the gap (top stitch or oversew.) Make the eyes with scraps of felt, or embroider them. Sew on one button and make a buttonhole to match. Make the next segment the same way, except that it will have *two* buttons and a button hole. Repeat the process all the way down, remembering to adjust the the buttonholes if the buttons vary in size.

Note

If you like your snake and plan to go into production, here is a useful tip for keeping the templates as a set. Punch a hole in each one and string them all together like beads on a necklace. I use a long piece of string for the 'necklace' and tie the ends together. When a pattern piece is needed, each one can easily be separated from its neighbours without untying the string.

TOYS USING OTHER FASTENINGS

An Australian Cushion

Quick

Take a tip from the Handbook of the Australian Association of Toy Libraries and make a special cushion covered with a variety of fastenings. Use the zip from an old pair of trousers; buttons and buttonholes from the front of a discarded dress; lacing holes cut from a worn-out canvas shoe (with laces) ; and find an old belt with a buckle. Sew them all firmly to a washable cushion cover. Put the cushion inside, and rest it on the table or the child's knee so that all the fastenings are within easy reach. Children react favourably to this trainer, because it uses items from real clothes. Maybe they will recognise the fancy buttons from the front of Auntie Mary's blouse!

Life-sized Baby Dolls

Long-lasting

Fran Whittle and
her team,
All Saints Arts and
Youth Centre,
Sussex

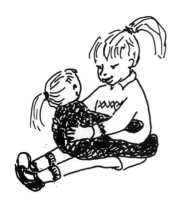

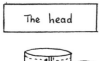

The head

Toys and trainers that help children to manipulate fastenings definitely have their uses, but they are no substitute for the real thing. Fran's dolls can be dressed in real hand-me-down clothes complete with zips, buttons, and Velcro—or even buckles, poppers and bows if the children can manage these.

Materials
- A Babygro, outgrown perhaps, or from the local jumble or car boot sale.
- Stretch fabric for the head. Fran recommends cotton stockinette.
- Polyester stuffing, with the CE safety mark on the pack.
- Wool, felt and thread for hair and features.

Method
First stuff the Babygro. Next make the head. Cut a strip of stretch fabric approximately right for the size of the Babygro. (A young baby's body is about 3½ times the length of its head, and its neck is very short.) Stitch the short sides of the strip together to make a ring of material. Run a thread along one edge, gather up and fasten off securely. This is the top of the head. Turn the material inside out. Run another thread around the open (neck) end, unthread the needle and leave the thread dangling. Stuff the head, re-thread the needle, draw up the running thread and again fasten off securely. Join the head to the top of the Babygro with several rounds of stitching. The doll will have a floppy head, just like a real baby. This makes it very appealing.

To make the face, first cut the features out of felt. Start with the eyes. These should be half way down the head (or slightly lower) and fairly wide apart. Pin them roughly in place. Do the same with the mouth (and nose?). Then try moving the pieces about a little to see how the expression changes. When you are satisfied, stitch the pieces in place and remove the pins. The hair can be made of wool. One method is to wind it over a piece of stiff paper and machine or hand sew it down the middle to keep the strands of wool in order. Cut the wool where it bends round the edges of the paper and tear the paper away. Consider the row of stitching to be the parting, and stitch the wool hair firmly to the head along this line. Trim off any straggly ends. Select some suitable clothes (with lots of fastenings on them!) from the 'cast offs', and your doll is ready for tender loving care!